# Dedication

To You My Dear Friends!

The Modern-Day Noah's Who Are Heeding the Word;

Building Your Ark of Protection and Health for the Great Nuclear and Cosmic Superstorm

# Special Mentions

**Dr. William Wong, Naturopathic Collaborator**

**Doug Diamond, Owner/Producer/Engineer, Diamondigital Media, Nashville, TN, 615-662-6870, doug@diamondiscaudio.com, www.diamondiscaudio.com**

**Dr. Philip Ranheim, my environmental medicine mentor**

**Steve Quayle, who graciously provides me a platform to get critical information to you! And**

**Shaunna Koblis, my friend, who stood by my side through my Moshe's cancer.  I was by her side with her Maggie's cancer.**

**David DuByne, ADAPT 2030, who faithfully informs the public on these topics in fascinating presentations!  Adapt 2030 YouTube Channel**

**Ben Davidson, Suspicious Observers, Space Weather Extraordinaire!**

# Table of Contents

# Electromagnetic Radiation Protection Solutions

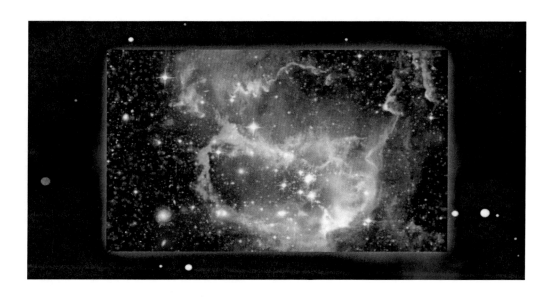

*God's Marvellous Protective Provisions*

*For the Nuclear & Solar Storm Crisis*

By

Celeste Solum

ISBN: 9781650061689

# Foreword

Welcome to my personal quest to unlock the mysteries of the invisible galactic cosmic rays and Solar Particle Event and soon coming nuclear crisis.

As wickedness abound upon the face of the earth the Lord in all His fury is beginning to rain celestial stones down upon mankind for his and her idolatry, following His Word. We are being bombarded by celestial dust, incoming asteroids, and meteors, with potential for cataclysmic comets. Civilization and empires have been annihilated and build up around these cyclical celestial events.

My journey began when I suddenly and unexpectedly broke six bones in several months which a shock because of my excellent diet and strenuous physical activity. As I was already writing about catastrophism, the Holy Spirit gently guided me to space weather, where I had that light bulb moment to inquire if cosmic rays might be a factor in my recent bone breakage. What I discovered is that a combination of incoming cosmic rays, the collapse of the earth's magnetosphere and the Eddy Grand Solar Minimum are all playing havoc with our bodies! As these events converge and intensify, our physical health and minds will degrade.

STOP! Take 3 minutes out of your busy day to survey your personal situation

Survey your body starting at your head and working down to your feet. Do you have pain? Do you have sudden or chronic health conditions in any part of your body? Do you have the stamina you desire for your age? Do you feel healthy? Do you look healthy? Do you have a healthy spiritual relationship with your Creator?

Do you have a healthy diet for your body style? Do you consume fast food or processed foods? How often? Do you eat foods laden with many chemicals either in production or to extend shelf life or adulterants?

What is the length of time between harvest of your food and consumption? Do you eat nutrient-dense foods? Do you consume GMO products?

Do you take nutritional supplements? Are you factoring in radio-protective supplements?

For those who believe in God, He provides a haven, just as he did for the Israelites during the Ten Plagues of Egypt. Together, we will explore this unique time in history and God's marvellous protective provisions for His people!

Is there any hope for mankind?

**Medical Disclaimer**

Due to current laws and regulations, all words in this book are labelled as:

*Artistic Entertainment*

## Medical Disclaimer

The information on this site is not intended or implied to be a substitute for professional medical advice, diagnosis or treatment. All content, including text, graphics, images, and information, contained on or available in this document is for general information purposes only. I make no representation and assumes no responsibility for the accuracy of information contained on or available through this web site, and such information is subject to change without notice. You are encouraged to confirm any information obtained from or through my research with other sources and review all information regarding any medical condition or treatment with your physician. NEVER DISREGARD PROFESSIONAL MEDICAL ADVICE OR DELAY SEEKING MEDICAL TREATMENT BECAUSE OF SOMETHING YOU HAVE READ ON OR ACCESSED.

I do not recommend, endorse or make any representation about the efficacy, appropriateness or suitability of any specific tests, products, procedures, treatments, services, opinions, health care providers or other information that may be contained on or available in this document. I AM NOT RESPONSIBLE, NOR LIABLE, FOR ANY ADVICE, COURSE OF TREATMENT, DIAGNOSIS OR ANY OTHER INFORMATION, SERVICES OR PRODUCTS THAT YOU OBTAIN THROUGH THIS DOCUMENT.

All information in this document has been extracted from both peer-review studies and white papers obtained from the National Institute of Health, NASA, and other agencies.

# Invisible Bombardment

I first became aware of invisible bombardment when my oldest child was born in the 1974. I had a beautiful and picture-perfect pregnancy. When my daughter was born, she had major birth defects. Her chance of survival was less than 5%. I beseeched the Lord for her survival, my prayers joining prayers being lifted up for her from Christian brothers and sisters around the world. It took a monumental effort, much like moving heaven and earth. She did survive and thrived.

Due to her unique cluster of mutations, we were invited to a conference of global physicians who had convened to discuss the effects of nuclear radiation. It was determined that she had been exposed to radiation early in my pregnancy. To my knowledge, I had experienced no radiological event, even though my husband was a submariner on a nuclear fast attack submarine.

Sometime in the 1990's, I learned the truth. I discovered that a nuclear submarine had been leaking radiation. Not only was my world turned upside down, but one-third of my Lamaze class had children with major birth defects.

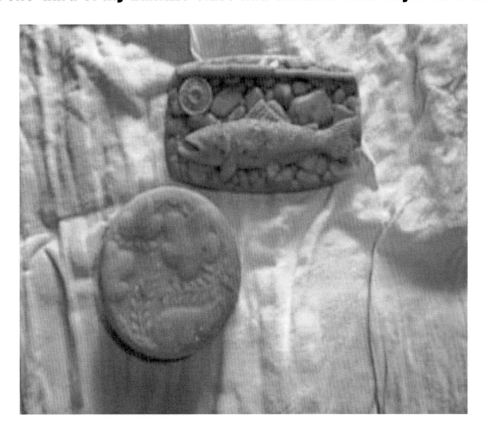

One month after Fukushima, in 2011, I had an unusual experience. As you know, I make soap, and I used to use chlorophyll to colour green soaps. To my shock as I was doing a presentation, I discovered that all my chlorophyll soaps had turned from green to a rusty orange.

The bible alludes to radiological events such as in Isaiah 17 and in Ezekiel during the Gog and Magog war. I wonder if when Jesus talked about wars and rumours of wars if He not only referred to known and unknown wars but also these invisible radiological wars that will surely significantly depopulates the planet.

You are not going to be told about many nuclear releases and our present cosmic superstorm of invisible bombardment by radioactive particles has been deliberately kept from you. Our planet has experienced these events in the past causing extinctions and mutations. According to most cultures and religions, this is the last cycle.

# Down and Dirty Bomb Protection from God

**We are all on budgets, but radioprotection does not need to break the bank. This is NASA's recommendation to its inner circle. This is not 100% protection, but each layer helps.**

• **Vitamin C**

• **N acetyl cycteine**

• **L-selenomethione (Selenium)**

• **Glutathione**

• **Lipolic Acid**

• **Vitamin E**

• **Dried Prunes or powered prunes (not fresh)**

# Preface

We have entered a galactic spiral arm that is inundating the earth with extraterrestrial dust while the earth's protective barrier, the magnetosphere, is collapsing, and our sun is going silent. This is a perfect storm of cosmic events that have caused species to go extinct, crushed civilizations, and destroyed empires. And yet it is only one small part of the catastrophism cycle that visits our planet periodically with varying intensity. As the very heavens are shaken, so too, is the earth convulsing as its foundations shake with earthquakes and violent eruptions of volcanism spewing ash into the stratosphere threatening to darken the sky and throw our globe into a Snowball planet.

At the beginning of the year, I began a book on Catastrophism to provide you with a comprehensive look at the back-story and how it will impact your life. I am well into my research, but I was impressed that you needed this information NOW! We are now at the beginning of this storm. You need to act. You will want to get your house in order. For some, it will be spiritual and others it will be physical, or a combination of both. There is a learning curve with this adaptation process. You might want to acquire certain supplies. I am noticing that certain supplies are disappearing from the shelves. You need to act now. I believe that I could not put your lives in peril to finish the more significant manuscript. What you are being presented are tools that are necessary for your survival.

I attempted to make it as user-friendly as I could. In the end, I left some medical terminology so that you can look things up on your own. I know it is dense, skim through parts that are not applicable. More importantly, I left medical terminology intact, so that you have a frank discussion with your medical provider about this imminent health threat. If you mention cosmic superstorm, you will get that deer-in-the-headlights look. But if you inquire about your specific health questions and personal situation providing peer-review and scientific evidence, your provider will take you more seriously. The cosmic and nuclear superstorm is not on the radar of your health care provider. There is going to be an exponential surge in deteriorating health issues and deaths. You do not want to be in that number.

This is your fleeting window of opportunity to build an ark of health.

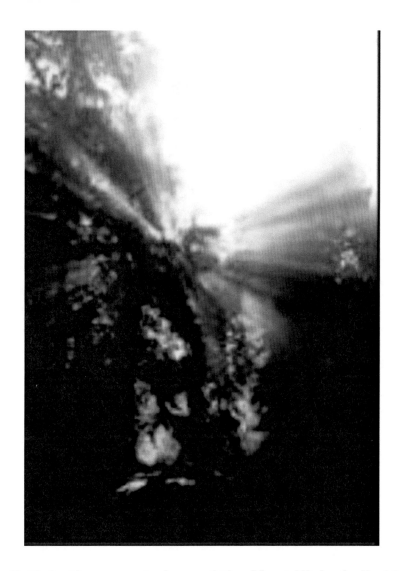

*He that dwelleth in the secret place of the Most High shall abide under the shadow of the Almighty. I will say of the LORD, He is my refuge and my fortress: my God; in him will I trust. Psalm 91*

# The Cosmic Ray

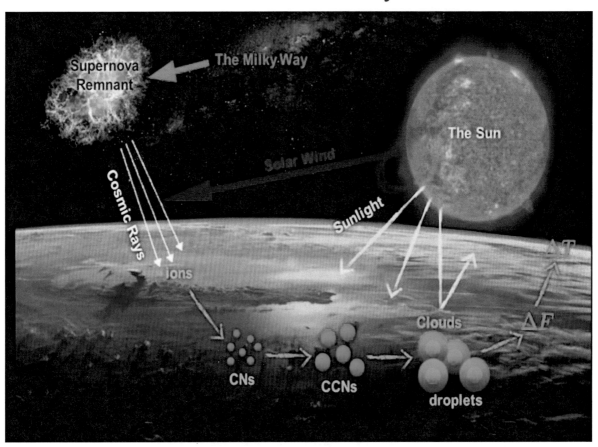

The Earth is protected against the cosmic radiation by its magnetosphere (magnetic field) and our atmosphere. Measurements of the Earth's magnetic field reveal a marked decrease over the Western hemisphere and increases over the Indian Ocean. There has been a general decrease in the magnetosphere intensity of 10% over the last 150 years. This decrease of the magnetosphere allows solar and galactic radioactive particles to reach the inner layers of the atmosphere. People at high altitudes or on-air flights are particularly vulnerable.

The Earth magnetosphere is a protective shield against solar flares that contain X-rays, and against the solar wind that transports electrons, protons, alpha particles, and heavier particles. The Sun's coronal mass ejections can carry ionized atomic matter with high kinetic energy, creating invisible shock waves allowing the fast-flowing particle to collisions, initiating the magnetic storms, through which, energetic ions and electrons can enter deep into the magnetic field, deep into the earth, and into all biological systems including your body.

The magnetosphere also provides earth with protection against galactic cosmic rays -a source of highly energetic particles with origin outside the solar system. These cosmic particles consist of different chemical elements, fully ionized.

During the intense solar activity, these cosmic particles are scattered by the solar wind, but when the Sun activity is reduced like it is currently (during the solar cycle), these cosmic particles slam into our atmosphere at high velocity and react with the atmospheric particles generating secondary particles that can reach the ground. The primary cosmic radiation has its origin from outside of our solar system, contains particles containing extremely high energy: Protons (10%), other heavier particles (These do not reach the sea level in the geographical areas that are protected by the strong magnetic field, but as our magnetosphere is collapsing they will be reaching earth.

Much like a billiard game, secondary cosmic radiation results from the interaction of the primary cosmic rays with the atmospheric particles, providing new particles of low energy.

# Up, Up and Away: The Cosmic Ray Threat

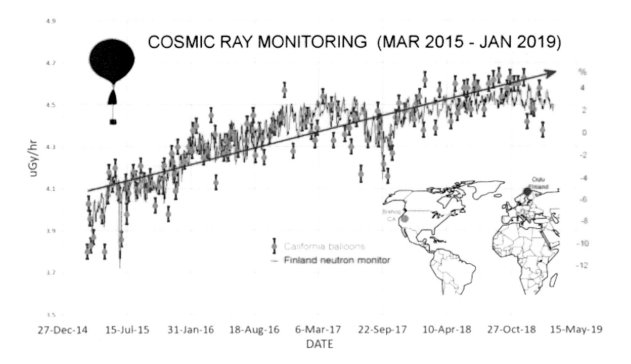

**Image: spaceweather.com**

**Key facts from the World Health Organization:**

• Ionizing radiation is a type of energy released by atoms in the form of electromagnetic waves or particles.

• People, animals, and plants are exposed to natural sources of ionizing radiation, such as in soil, water, and vegetation, as well as in human-made sources, such as x-rays and medical devices. Ionizing radiation is bio-accumulative, which means that it builds up in your body with continual exposure.

• As ionizing radiation increases, so does the potential for health hazards if not adequately addressed.

• Acute health effects such as skin burns or acute radiation syndrome can occur when doses of radiation exceed certain levels.

• Low doses of ionizing radiation can increase the risk of longer-term effects such as cancer.

# What is ionizing radiation?

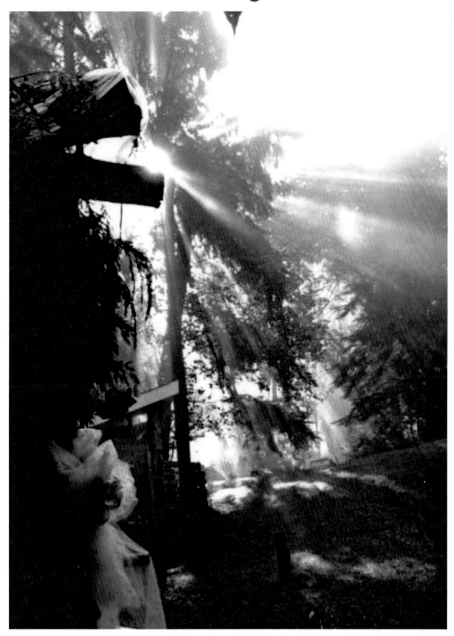

Ionizing radiation is a type of energy released by atoms that travel in the form of electromagnetic waves (gamma or X-rays) or particles (neutrons, beta, or alpha).

All radionuclides are uniquely identified by the type of radiation they emit, the energy of the radiation, and their half-life.

Your dosage of ionizing radiation will vary up to 200% depending upon where you live on the planet during exposure and your altitude.

# FAQ: Know Your Ionizing Radiation

## Alpha Radiation is also called alpha ray

Consisting of two protons and two neutrons bound together into a particle identical to a helium-4 nucleus. These particles have a low-penetration depth, so they remain blocked in the skin, where they can produce persistent oxidative stress. They are generally produced in the process of alpha decay but may also be produced in other ways. The symbol for Alpha particles comes from the Greek alphabet, a.

## Celestial Dust:

In a celestial dust assessment by Dr. Chiu Wing Lam identified that even impact exposure to dust from extra-terrestrial sources: can range from being a minor nuisance to having significant health implications. These specks of dust can have a high content of respirable size particles, have large surface areas that are chemically reactive, and contain nanoparticles of highly-reactive elements, like iron,- mixing with ubiquitous engineered nanoparticle saturation particles creating a synergistic effect. The unusual properties may cause the respirable dust to be moderately toxic to the respiratory system and the larger grains to be abrasive to the skin and eyes. There is a possibility that exposure to this dust can lead to dangerous respiratory, cardiopulmonary, ocular, central nervous system (CNS), or dermal harm.

## Electrons:

Electrons are subatomic particles, whose electric is negative one elementary charge. Electrons are leptons.

## Gamma Rays or gamma radiation (symbol $\gamma$)

Have the smallest wavelengths, penetrating, and the most energy of any other wave in the electromagnetic spectrum. Gamma-rays can kill living cells. The radiation stimulates nitric oxide synthesis in the cells, especially in the brain, liver, small intestine and colon. It increases the lipids, proteins, vitamin C, and folate oxidation.

**HZE** are highly charged energy particles.

**56Fe ions** are a dense iron nucleus particle from a galactic cosmic ray.

## Galactic Cosmic Rays

**Galactic cosmic rays are a form of high-energy radiation, mainly originating outside the Solar System and even from distant galaxies.**

## Muons:

**Muons (from the Greek letter mu (µ) used to represent it) is an elementary particle like the electron, with an electric charge of -1 e and a spin of 1/2, but with a much higher mass. It is a lepton.**

## Neutrons:

**A subatomic particle with an atomic nucleus with a mass of one and a charge of zero. Neutrons can transfer their energy to the hydrogen atoms located in your body tissues and produce recoil protons that can damage your bodily tissues. Protons and neutrons constitute the nuclei of atoms.**

## Photons:

**Photons are a type of elementary particle, the quantum of the electromagnetic field, including electromagnetic radiation such as light, radio waves, and the force carrier for the electromagnetic force-static or virtual particles.**

## Solar Particle Event (SPE) is a cosmic proton event or "proton storm." It

**occurs when particles (mostly protons.) emitted by the Sun become accelerated during a solar flare or by Coronal Mass Ejections (CME) shocks. The events can include other nuclei such as helium ions and HZE ions, causing multiple effects to the body.**

## X-rays make up X-radiation,

**a form of high-energy electromagnetic radiation. X-rays are a form of electromagnetic radiation that is used for medical imaging, treating cancer, and even used for exploring the cosmos... They can cause DNA alterations and release electrons with an energy capable of ionizing your body, causing tissue damage. X-rays decrease the levels of Vitamin C and Vitamin E in your body.**

# Cosmic Ray Exposure Health Effects

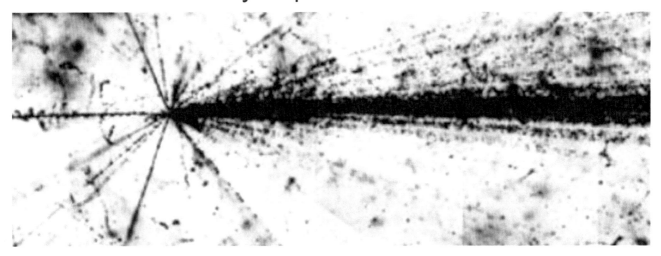

The radiation spectrum of cosmic radiation contains different particles with a broad range of energies that can produce different effects on the human body. Radiation produces:

• Immediate results causing DNA damage, signal scrambling, break bonds, and .,

• Early results are demonstrated in DNA repair, mutation, genomic instability, induced gene expression, cell cycle perturbation, and apoptosis.

• Late effects include altered functions of the body's systems, cataracts, and cancer.

Radiation effects on the body's cells can be caused by direct action to the DNA and indirect action through the reactive oxygen and nitrogen species or by the alterations of other cellular molecules. The oxidative stress initiated by the ionizing radiation is responsible for two-thirds of DNA damages. To give you an example, mice irradiated with protons had reduced leukocyte's number. They still had oxidative stress that altered the stem cells in their bone marrow a full two months after exposure.

Degenerative tissue risks include adverse radiation biologic effects on the heart, circulatory, endocrine, digestive, lens, and other tissue systems (which would consist of radiation effects on bone, muscle, etc.). This is what piqued my interest in this topic. I broke six bones in 3 months, despite a very healthy diet and vigorous exercise, which piqued my curiosity as to why. My healthy dog also collapsed and died with 21 days of hemangiosarcoma.

Radiation exposure may be internal or external and can be acquired through various exposure pathways. Although you can be exposed to ionizing radiation from many sources, for the purposes of this document, we will be discussing primarily galactic cosmic, solar rays, and to some degree, nuclear radiation.

Internal exposure to ionizing radiation occurs when a radionuclide is inhaled, ingested, or otherwise enters the bloodstream through wounds and other entryways. Internal exposure stops when the radionuclide is eliminated from the body, either spontaneously (such as through excreta) or as a result of treatment.

External exposure may occur when airborne radioactive materials (such as dust, liquid, or aerosols) are deposited on skin or clothes which can remove by washing.

NASA did an assessment of risks related to exposure to solar particle event (SPE) radiation breaking the damage down into four categories.

• Acute and Late Central Nervous System Effects,

• Acute Radiation Syndromes Due to Solar Particle Events (SPEs),

• Degenerative Tissue or other Health Effects from Radiation Exposure,

• Risk of Radiation Cancer (Just in! 2019-cancer will rise exponentially)

# Stages of Ionizing Radiation Exposure

Stages of exposure exposed to ionizing radiation you go through different stages:

1. The PRODROMAL PHASE, which commences during the initial period (within an hour to around a day) after the exposure. This is an acute (immediate medical condition);

2. The LATENT PHASE, the duration of which depends on the intensity of exposure; and

3. The ILLNESS PHASE, which has the characteristic features of the syndrome bearing its name. This frequently becomes a chronic medical condition until resolution.

4. The RECOVERY or DEATH PHASE

In the first **PRODROMAL PHASE**, you begin to experience symptoms such as nausea, vomiting, malaise, and myalgia (body aches). The time to onset of nausea and vomiting correlates directly with the radiation dose that the individual is exposed to.

During the **LATENT PHASE**, you may remain relatively symptom-free. The length of the latent phase varies from hours to even a month, depending on the intensity of radiation exposure. GI syndromes can last days to a week while neurovascular (blood vessels in the brain) just a few hours.

The **ILLNESS PHASE** appears with the classical clinical symptoms associated with the primary organ system that has been injured (bone marrow, intestine, or neurovascular effects).

The **RECOVERY or DEATH PHASE** is self-explanatory. The victim will either recovery gradually or die.

# Radiation Relevant Medical Glossary

## Apoptosis

**is programmed cell death from a Greek word meaning "falling off," as leaves from a tree.**

## Gastrointestinal tract bacterial translocation

**bacteria permeate through your gut wall into your body.**

## Lipid peroxidation

**Lipid peroxidation is the oxidative degradation of lipids. It is the process in which free radicals "steal" electrons from the lipids in cell membranes, resulting in cell damage.**

## Oxidation

**A chemical reaction in which reactant combines with oxygen or loses hydrogen to form the product is called an oxidation reaction. Think of it as biological rust.**

## Peripheral hematopoietic stem cells-

**These are your immature stem cells that can form into any cell in your body. They take 6-8 weeks to mature. If they encounter something such as an allergen or ionizing radiation, they become permanently damaged. Your body is continuously making new stem cells, so it continually has an opportunity to heal if the offending exposure ceases. Indeed you are a new creation!**

## Pharmacokinetics (PK)

**is defined as the study of the time course of drug absorption, distribution, metabolism, and excretion; clinical pharmacokinetics is the application of pharmacokinetic principles for safe and effective therapeutic management of patients.**

## Pharmacodynamics (PD)

**refers to the relationship between drug concentration at the site of action and the resulting effect, including the time course and intensity of therapeutic and adverse effects.**

## Reactive Species:

**A type of unstable molecule that contains oxygen and that quickly reacts with other molecules in a cell. A build-up of reactive oxygen species in cells may**

cause damage to DNA, RNA, and proteins, and may cause cell death. Reactive oxygen species are free radicals.

# Radiation and Your Body

High-energy electrons exposure leads to protein damage in living organisms.

Most low-energy electrons of cosmic origin are absorbed within the skin, particularly the epidermis and partially within the dermis.

Ionizing radiation causes DNA lesions by direct action or indirect action, through the increased concentration of reactive species that are generated. This persists for weeks after radiation exposure.

The reactive species that are produced can be neutralized by the scavengers. Superoxide and hydrogen peroxide are relatively stable, so they persist in the tissue for more extended periods. They can diffuse and continue the oxidative stress into the deeper tissues, causing DNA damages, protein oxidation, and lipid peroxidation.

Irradiated cells produce an intercellular communication that continues the damages into the body through reactive oxygen species, cytokines, RNAs, or calcium ions, molecules that are released and received by the distant cells that were not irradiated.

Increased cosmic rays (CR) exposure can stimulate the activity of the parasympathetic system. The effects of cosmic radiation on the cardiovascular system are the directly proportional relationship between cosmic radiation activity and monthly death numbers. The increased activity of CR affects the electrical activity of the heart and can disturb the lipid metabolism in the artery wall. Neutrons enter the body and are converted to protons in the tissues with a high content of H+ ions (including atheroma). The protons can destroy the cells leading to fatal arrhythmia in ischaemic cardiomyopathy, acute myocardial infarction (heart attack), and can produce atheroma ruptures formation of the lumen (kind of plaque-like blockages that rupture). McCraty et al.

Cosmic ray's exposure affects the visual system. In the eye, cosmic radiation initiates a chain reaction that generates different reactive species and photons, explaining light flashes and other visual experiences.

Radiation damage to tissue and/or organs depends on the dose of radiation received or the absorbed dose, which is expressed in a unit called the gray (Gy). The potential damage from an absorbed dose depends on the type of radiation and the sensitivity of different tissues and organs.

Beyond certain thresholds, radiation can impair the functioning of tissues and/or organs and can produce acute effects such as skin redness, hair loss, radiation burns, or acute radiation syndrome. These effects are more severe at higher doses and higher dose rates. The dose threshold for acute radiation syndrome is about 1 Sv.

If the radiation dose is low and/or it is delivered over a long period (low dose rate), the risk is substantially lower because your body can repair the damage. There is still a risk of long-term effects such as cancer, even decades later. Outcomes of this type will not always occur, but their likelihood is proportional to the radiation dose. This risk is higher for children and adolescents, as they are significantly more sensitive to radiation exposure than adults.

Epidemiological studies on populations exposed to radiation, such as atomic bomb survivors, showed a significant increase in cancer risk at doses above 100 mSv. More recently, some epidemiological studies in individuals exposed to medical exposures during childhood suggested that cancer risk may increase even at lower doses (between 50-100 mSv).

Prenatal exposure to ionizing radiation may induce brain damage in fetuses following an acute dose exceeding 100 mSv between weeks 8-15 of pregnancy and 200 mSv between weeks 16-25 of pregnancy. Before week 8 or after week 25 of a human pregnancy, studies have not shown radiation risk to fetal brain development.

# Cardiovascular Disease and Other Degenerative Tissue Effects from Radiation Exposure and Secondary Stressors

Exposure to ionizing radiation from such as gamma and x-rays, either from a nuclear event or cosmic superstorms including solar particle events (SPE) cause many degenerative tissues (non-cancer) adverse health issues including diseases in:

- Cardiovascular (heart),

- Cerebrovascular (brain),

- Cataracts,

- Accelerated aging,

- Digestive disorders

- Endocrine (hormone) disorders,

- Immune system failure or activation,

- Respiratory dysfunction

Cardiovascular pathologies such as atherosclerosis (hardening of the arteries) and cerebrovascular (stroke) disease are of significant concern following gamma-ray exposure such as the during the coronal hole plasma waves frequently streaming to earth.

Scientists in cross-disciplinary collaboration are attempting to discover what the low-dose thresholds are for a human, the impact of dose-rate, and radiation quality effects, as well as mechanisms and pathways; are not well-characterized.

Degenerative disease risks are often difficult to assess because of multiple factors, including radiation. They are believed to play a role in the etiology of many diseases. For instance, lifestyle choices such as obesity, alcohol, improper nutrition, and tobacco use can lead to similar adverse outcomes, clouding population-based risk models, and contributing to the significant uncertainties.

We are the guinea pigs in a massive radiological experiment. Ubiquitous sensors are documenting the real-time effects of ionizing radiation on humans, animals, and plant life. Policymakers are in the process of developing a Permissible Exposure Limits (PELs). This will quantify the impact on disease-free survival years after you are exposed, not so much for you, but to know when you will die. The possibility of radiation exposure interacting with other secondary stressors is also being evaluated.

# Acute Radiation Syndromes from
## Solar Particle Events (SPE's)

A variety of acute radiation syndromes are of concern following a large nuclear or SPE, including radiation sicknesses, nausea, vomiting, diarrhea, and fatigue. These effects are manifested within 4 to 24 hours post-exposure for sub-lethal doses, with a latency time inversely correlated with dose. There is a reasonable concern for a compromised immune system due to high skin doses after a nuclear or SPE event. There is a remote possibility of acute death through the collapse of the blood-forming systems.

The effects related to various types of nuclear and space radiation exposures that have been evaluated thus far are:

• **DNA changes and mutations**

• **Gene Expression Changes. This could alter your epigenetic expression originating in your RNA, primarily associated with programmed cell death known as apoptosis (programmed cell death from a Greek word meaning "falling off," as leaves from a tree) and extracellular matrix (ECM) remodeling or restructuring),**

• **Increased oxidative stress- Oxidative stress is essentially an imbalance between the production of free radicals and the ability of the body to counteract or detoxify.**

• **Gastrointestinal tract bacterial translocation-where bacteria permeate through your gut wall into your body.**

• **Immune system activation- The innate immune system is made of defenses against infection that can be activated immediately once a pathogen attack. It can be useful when fighting harmful bacteria, although bad when the immune system against itself, as in the case of auto-immune diseases.**

• **Destroys or mutates peripheral hematopoietic cell counts- These are your immature stem cells that can form into any cell in your body. They take 6-8 weeks to mature. If they encounter something such as an allergen or ionizing radiation, they become permanently damaged. Your body is continually making new stem cells, so it frequently has an opportunity to heal if the offending exposure ceases. Indeed you are a new creation!**

- Emesis is vomiting

- Blood coagulation is known as your blood clotting factor.

- Skin integrity

- Behavior/fatigue (social exploration, exercise spontaneous locomotor activity),

- Heart and brain functions

- Alterations in vision

- Alterations in taste (taste aversion)

- Cancer, Survival

- Cataract development-this can come on in mere days

# Cardiovascular (Heart) System

Cardiac arrhythmia (irregular heartbeat) can often be attributed to a cosmic superstorm. Factors such as age and sex, as well as cardiovascular risk factors and pre-existing arrhythmias, are likely contributing to arrhythmia, but it is unclear whether stressors potentate the risk.

Exposure to some elements such as radiation, physical and psychological stress, altered diet, and exercise habits may exacerbate the risk of heart rhythm disturbances. Some arrhythmias, such as atrial fibrillation, can develop over time, necessitating periodic screening.

The heart and circulatory effects resulting from exposure to ionizing radiations have recently been reported that doses of 2 to 5 Gy 56Fe ion radiation targeted to specific arterial sites in mice accelerate the development of atherosclerosis (hardening of the arteries). In these studies, it was concluded that 56Fe ions can promote the progression of atherosclerotic lesions to an advanced stage characterized by compositional changes indicative of increased thrombogenicity (blood clot) and instability.

# Renal-Kidney System

It is important to note that renal stone formation (kidney stones) can occur within the renal-kidney system after irradiation.

Ensure that you maintain a quality dietary and appropriate fluid intake to positively influence your urine pH and fluid volume to avoid adverse renal-kidney system issues, including kidney stones.

# Acute & Late Central Nervous System Effects from Radiation Exposure

Current research is ongoing to establish possible threshold doses for specific central nervous risks (CNS) risks from galactic cosmic rays (GCR) is a concern. This is due to the possibility of single high charge and energy (HZE) nuclei traversals causing tissue damage, as evidenced by the light-flash phenomenon first observed during the Apollo missions. This can and will happen on earth as well.

Cancer patients have shown persistent CNS changes long after treatment with gamma rays suggesting a possible CNS risk for a significant solar particle event (SPE). Furthermore, animal studies of behavior and performance with HZE radiation suggest detrimental changes may occur during long-term GCR exposures. Currently, there is no projection model for CNS risks of concern to NASA.

Exposure to low doses of space radiation of Gamma Rays ($\gamma$-rays) or Iron ($^{56}Fe$) ions is known to have adverse effects on CNS and neuro-behavior in irradiated humans and animals, including:

• Reduced performance in motor tasks

• Deficits in spatial learning and memory

Alterations in neuronal function after HZE particle exposure include increased Nigral cell loss in your brain, which parallel the neurobehavioral changes associated with aging and Parkinsonism.

# Sticks and Stones Can Break Your Bones (And Skeleton),

## So, Can A Nuclear or Cosmic Superstorm!

Bone atrophy is targeted to specific regions of the skeleton. While we will not experience the minimal gravity that astronauts experience, the earth, and cosmic changes can influence our bones. In space, the average decrement of pre-flight areal bone mineral density (BMD) per month is 1-1.5%,

It is important to remember this unique time in history:

• Bone changes occur

• Multiple factors during our current environment, both space, and earth, can influence bone changes.

• The relative contribution of microarchitecture and bone geometry to whole bone strength is not known.

• Due to the multiple contributors to bone strength, the full-on overall bone strength is unknown.

# Risk of Early Onset Osteoporosis

The fracture and bone risks are interrelated because they have the same physiological outcome—bone fracture. In my research, I discovered that our bones could become vulnerable and subject to fracture with as little as two weeks of irradiation. The good news is that proactively consuming some of the protective provisions, your bones strengthen, in just two weeks!

However, the risks differ regarding the type, cause, and timing of fracture, and the mitigation approach and resources. The descriptions of skeletal changes will inform both risks. The crux of managing both risks depends on the ability to estimate when fractures will likely occur.

Osteoporosis is a condition of low mass and microarchitectural disruptions in the bone that increases the risk of fragility fractures, i.e., fractures that can occur with little or no applied loads. Osteoporosis typically manifests in geriatrics (older people) because it is often the result of slow, chronic bone loss due to aging.

It is possible that bone can atrophy requiring mitigation to prevent fractures, but scientists have not yet determined bone changes or individual susceptibility to multiple risk factors that are needed to determine the individual probability of bone fracture. Policymakers for age-related osteoporosis and bone densitometry suggest that these standards are not useful for assessing skeletal integrity in an exposure. The overarching approach to address the osteo risk with advanced surveillance.

Irradiation with gamma-rays exacerbates skeletal microarchitectural changes that are usually found during the progressive onset of age-related osteoporosis. Radiation exposure increases reactive oxygen species production and oxidative damage, which implies different molecular mechanisms from the bone loss caused by disuse.

Irradiation with 250 MeV protons results in loss of the bone volume fraction and connectivity density. Whole, irradiation with iron 56 Fe ions, which represents a significant component of galactic cosmic rays (GCR), enhances the sensitivity of bone cells to the effects of radiation.

Iron ion radiation contributes to a reduction in adaptive responses to your back. Thus, irradiation with heavy ions may accelerate or worsen the loss of skeletal integrity triggered by musculoskeletal disuse, as in the case of winter confinement or other factors that promote a sedentary lifestyle.

# Cognitive or Behavioural Conditions and Psychiatric Disorders

You must become aware that SPE, cosmic superstorm, or nuclear event can trigger a variety of cognitive, behavioral, or psychiatric conditions. Yes, it is true; I even am noticing this in my own body.

Central Nervous System (CNS), Sensorimotor (CBS) Integrated Research Plan identified four risks:

• Risk of Acute and Late Central Nervous System Effects from Radiation Exposure Acronym is CNS

• Risk of Adverse Cognitive or Behavioural Conditions and Psychiatric Disorders Acronym is BMed

• Risk of Impaired control of mechanical and craft such as vehicles/associated systems and decreased mobility due to vestibular/sensorimotor alterations

• Risk of Inadequate Human-Computer Interaction and situational awareness

Our information displays must be designed with a fully developed operational concept, fine-grained task analysis, and knowledge of human information processing capabilities and limitations, the format, mode, and layout of the information may not optimally support task performance. Otherwise, it may result in users misinterpreting, overlooking, or ignoring the original intent of the information, leading to task completion times that impact the timeline, necessitating costly re-planning and rescheduling, and/or task execution errors, which endanger your mission, safety, and mission success.

Situation awareness (SA) is also a critical factor in the execution of tasks. SA refers to the perception of environmental elements concerning time and/or space, the comprehension of their meaning, and the projection of their status after something has changed, such as time. You must be able to perceive relevant changes in those displays (e.g., component temperature rising), comprehend what that means in context (e.g., component approaching upper-temperature threshold/overheating), and be able to predict what may happen next. During this pivotal time in history, this type of situation awareness must be maintained for a multitude of variables across multiple spectrums at lightning speed.

# Low Oxygen

## Risk of Reduced Health and Performance Due to Hypoxia

Believe it or not, geoengineering is not only taking carbon dioxide out of our atmosphere but also oxygen! That is what we breathe-to live!

A decreased level of oxygen in the body's organs and systems affects all physiological functions. Supposedly, it is said to induce only mild hypoxic stress, which healthy individuals can tolerate well on Earth. For example, millions of people live at altitudes higher than 4000 ft. Even more, people experience mild transient hypoxia during airplane flights at 5000-8000 ft.

But the truth is very different.

The first number will be oxygen concentration percentage and the second symptoms of a person at rest

19% Some adverse physiological effects can occur, but they may not be noticeable.

15-19% Impaired thinking and attention. Increased pulse and breathing rate. Decreased ability to work strenuously. Reduced physical and intellectual performance.   Intellectual performance awareness-can you say, zombie?

12-15% Poor judgment. Faulty coordination. Abnormal fatigue upon exertion. Emotional upset.

10-12% Inferior judgment and coordination. Also, impaired respiration may cause permanent heart damage. Possibility of fainting within a few minutes without warning. Nausea and vomiting.

<10 Inability to move. Fainting almost immediate. Loss of consciousness. Convulsions. Death

# Sleep and Circadian System

## Risk of Performance Decrements and Adverse Health Outcomes Resulting from Sleep Loss, Circadian Desynchronization, and Work Overload

If you struggle with insomnia, brace yourself for the cosmic superstorm, because sleep is reduced, and circadian rhythms are misaligned. I have personally experienced this less than favorable impact as waves of particles hit the earth.

Studies indicate that adequately timed light exposure can help maintain circadian alignment and/or facilitate schedule shifting, performance, and alertness. You may have to limit screen time near bedtime and resort to herbal supplements.

As prophetic and cyclical events unfold, our workload is inevitably going to get strenuous. For some, this may be physical labor, others mental, while others exertion in the supernatural realm such as prayer. Whatever your calling or job- is about to explode, requiring massive amounts of time and energy. This creates work overload.

# Social Interaction

## Risk of Performance and Behavioural Health Decrements Due to Inadequate Cooperation, Coordination, Communication, and Psychosocial Adaptation within a Team

As noted in Chan Thomas's, Adam and Eve Story, as we enter the cosmic superstorm or experience a nuclear event, a cascade-disintegration occurs disrupting:

• Cooperation

• Coordination

• Communication

• Psychosocial Adaptation

The government and the military are aware that this set of environmental factors will increase violence. This is going to impact your family, community, faith community, country and the world at large. Pay attention to space weather in the coming days, months, and years, and you will notice these trends. With this understanding, you can better manage your situation and extend extra grace and patience to others.

Remember that as the fabric of society changes with wickedness and violence increasing due to environmental factors, we might be faced with the possibility of relocation (refugee). The record of history demonstrates that the plight of a refugee is not always favorable, especially as certain elements restructure our world. You may discover yourself forming new networks, but the question is, how cohesive will they be due to this social interaction dimension of the cosmic superstorm and/or nuclear event?

# Inadequate Nutrition

Nutrition will be critical to your success in your path of faith during a long duration of a physically and spiritually harsh environment. Nutrition will be an essential countermeasure for maintaining your health.

Your food preps during the famine must be palatable, enjoyable, and chemically stable for the duration of the famine to ensure they meet the nutritional needs. A limited variety of food and the repetition of menu cycles could lead to reduced intake and inadequate nutrition. Understand that people who consume fast foods or highly processed foods will die first. You must also factor in the United Nations food control system that is in effect as I pen this manuscript.

The most basic role of food and nutrition is to prevent nutrient deficiency during stressful events such as famine. The typical western diet is still limited in some nutrients. Individuals who restrict their intake of certain foods or food categories increase their risk of nutrient deficiencies—for example,

• Vegetarians need to be mindful of meeting protein, iron, and Vitamin B12 requirements;

• People who avoid fruits and vegetables are at higher risk of vitamin deficiencies;

• Individuals who are trying to lose weight by reducing calories or following defined diet protocols have deficiencies in specific micronutrients.

As the Eddy Grand Solar Minimum dawns, we must be well-nourished before and during this critical time. While preventing nutrient deficits is crucial, optimizing nutrition will maintain health and enable your spiritual race success. We know much less about the effects of diet and nutrition on performance than we do about how to prevent nutrient deficiency. We must learn how food and nutrition interact with the human system to optimize health and performance. This becomes even more critical in a cosmic superstorm situation where environmental factors like radiation and stress can all affect nutrient metabolism, physiology and biochemistry, and health and performance. Optimized food provisions will protect you against many of the physiological impacts including ophthalmic, cardiovascular, musculoskeletal, immunological, and radiation-induced effects. Nutrition also includes adequate fluid intake to maintain hydration and minimize kidney stones. Food choices and nutritional status are known to affect performance and cohesion. Nutrition enables optimal exercise performance and has documented effects on circadian rhythms and sleep. Food and nutrition are obvious behavior/performance countermeasures. Food choices (e.g., fruit and vegetable intake) and nutritional status are known effectors on performance and cohesion.

Cardiovascular and ophthalmologic issues, bone and muscle loss, response to exercise, and even the effects of environmental exposures (radiation, oxygen, and carbon dioxide) all interact with nutrition. We must understand the acute and chronic effects of these interactions. Fruit and vegetable intake are critically limited in the current food supply. Fruit and vegetable intake are associated with mood, cognition, behavior, and performance, and has beneficial effects on cardiovascular, immune, bone, muscle, and antioxidant protection systems. The food system is very limited in sources of Omega-3 Fatty Acids- healthy fats that have been shown to improve cardiovascular health on Earth and are also associated with improved bone health.

Increased iron from incoming iron cosmic ray particles is associated with increased oxidative damage to your DNA and is also correlated with bone loss. Nutrition can offset high levels of urinary calcium resulting from bone loss from these cosmic ray events.

We have a choice. We can do as some ship captains did centuries ago, denying the reports of the effects of citrus fruit, and argue instead that clean galleys and fresh meat would eradicate scurvy. Or, we can optimize nutrition and our health during these trying times, helping to ensure that our race is finished well while imparting long-lasting benefits on our physical health

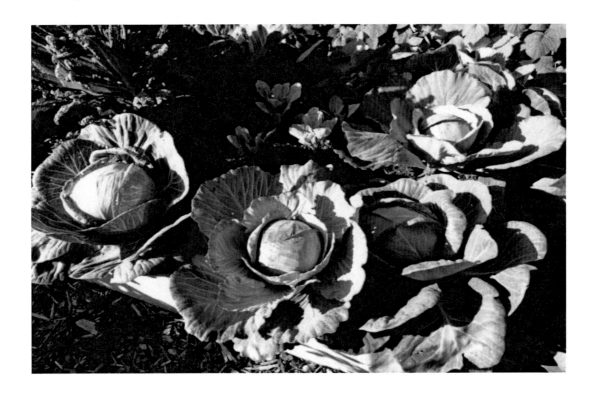

# Immune System

## Risk of Adverse Health Event Due to Altered Immune Response

In a cosmic superstorm or nuclear event, not to mention the ongoing collapse of the magnetosphere, our cells are going to go haywire because they will have difficulty in communicating and doing their jobs.

Recent investigations have found that certain aspects of immunity are dysregulated can persist. It appears that specific adverse medical symptoms occur in select people (and yes, they know who those people are) – including atypical allergic symptoms, atopic dermatitis, or various infectious processes – may relate to immune dysregulation.

Immune dysregulation is likely to worsen due to the synergistic factor with increased levels of radiation exposure, stress, and circadian misalignment. The immune system is complicated, consisting of many distinct types of cells, each with a unique function.

Exposure to proton radiation represents the significant type of radiation in Solar Particle Events (SPE). It is known to induce abnormalities in your blood, including your leukocytes, erythrocytes, and platelets, along with reasonable concern for compromised immune functions.

The consistent effects on the immune system observed are as follows: reduction in peripheral T-cell counts and a decrease in Natural Killer (NK), cell number, and functionality. Numerous immune system alterations can occur. This medical terminology will provide you an indication of what can go wrong-feel free to speed read or scan. I include this for a medical professional attending to your health needs during these events:

There are changes in cytokine production, leukocyte subset distribution, and antibody production. Examples of cytokines released in response to stimulation include the following: an increase in anti-inflammatory cytokines and a decrease in TNF-a in LPS stimulated spleen cells, reductions in interferon-$\gamma$, and IL-2 following phorbol 12-myristate 13-acetate and ionomycin stimulation of peripheral blood cells and reduced NK cell number and function. Such alterations in immune function are like those brought about when there is increased immune activation produced by exposure to pathogen-associated molecular patterns (PAMPs), such as LPS. Specific examples of this are as follows: a reduction in proinflammatory cytokine production by myeloid cells, a decrease in antigen-specific T cell effector cytokine responses, and a reduction in circulating NK cells. The changes in reactions brought about by exposure to PAMPs are known as "tolerance," in which subsequent responses are reduced in quality and quantity, which is thought to protect the host by limiting excessive inflammation and preventing septic shock. As has been observed in many different disease states, continuous or extended exposure to PAMPs can lead to long-lived immune dysfunction. This condition may exist during space flight and increasingly on earth, as LBP, a well-known marker of immune activation, is known to be elevated in astronauts' plasma. The elevated blood levels of LBP resulting from exposure to SPE radiation and simulated microgravity (HS) may bring about immune dysfunctions of the sort that have been observed during and after extended spaceflight.

# Adverse Health Effects Due to Host-Microorganism Interactions

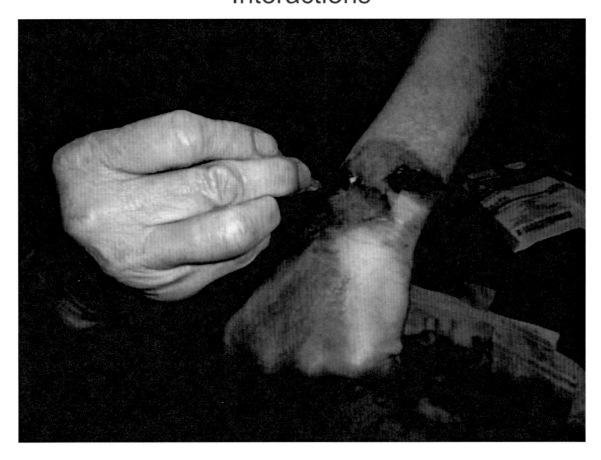

Despite the United Nations' grand effort to eradicate pathogens (infections), they are a part of life and here to stay. There is evidence which indicates that specific characteristics of microorganisms are altered when microbes are exposed to cosmic rays. These alterations include changes in virulence (disease-causing potential). This is your super-pandemic warning!

## Unpredicted Effects of Medication

If you take any type of medication or during this cosmic or nuclear superstorm, you need to be aware that your drugs and supplements are going to behave differently in your body. It might be attributed to the cellular activity or that your microbiome (gut) is out of whack. The way you metabolize medications and supplements is going to change. This alteration can cause you to become symptomatic. For instance, I noticed that my regular supplementation was not working any longer. I experimented a bit and discovered, personally, that I needed to increase my intake seven-fold, but within recommended allowances. Never increase dosages without consulting a health care practitioner.

This comes to you from NASA: Pharmacokinetics (PK) is defined as the study of the time course of drug absorption, distribution, metabolism, and excretion; clinical pharmacokinetics is the application of pharmacokinetic principles for safe and effective therapeutic management of patients. The primary goals of clinical pharmacokinetics are enhancing drug efficacy and decreasing drug toxicity. Pharmacodynamics (PD) refers to the relationship between drug concentration at the site of action and the resulting effect, including the time course and intensity of therapeutic and adverse effects. Combining knowledge of drug potency, PK, and PD enables us to assess the efficacy and safety of medications.

Because of the physiological changes that occur, it seems likely that pharmacokinetics (PK) (how the body handles administered medication) and possibly pharmacodynamics (PD) (how the administered drug affects the body) could be different. Knowledge of medication use, efficacy, and side effects are expected to provide preliminary information on these points.

## Sensory and Endurance

### Risk of Impaired Control and Decreased Mobility Due to Vestibular/Sensorimotor Alterations

Our changing magnetosphere can induce adaptive central reinterpretation of visual, vestibular, and proprioceptive information. These changes are most prevalent during and after transitions and lead to performance. During adaptation and re-adaptation periods, disturbances in perception, spatial orientation, posture, gait, eye-head, and eye-head-hand coordination occur that disrupt a person's ability to control vehicles and complex systems and to move around and perform tasks. Due to a number changes your perception of things like taste aversion and "seeing things."

## Impaired Performance Due to Reduced Muscle Mass, Strength & Endurance and Reduced Aerobic Capacity

Space travel is known to diminish muscle mass, strength, and aerobic capacity. You can also experience it on earth as environmental and social conditions require us to shelter-in-place at home. Many of us may see the day we become refugees within our own homes. The day this happens, whether it is from bad weather or violence, the risk of impaired physical performance increases due to reduced muscle mass, strength, and endurance and reduced aerobic capacity.

Effective exercise countermeasures are the primary strategies to mitigate the risks.

Sensorimotor and neuro vestibular impairments also contribute to reduced physical performance. Loss of aerobic fitness and muscle size and strength are normal physiological responses to being kept indoors for lengthy periods due to hostile environmental conditions.

For instance, astronauts lose an average of 17% of their maximal aerobic capacity (VO2pk) within the first two weeks of spaceflight. Astronauts lose an average of 5-20% of their pre-flight upper and lower leg muscle strength during spaceflight. This can happen to you when you retreat to your bug out spot or home for extended periods.

# Risk of Associated Neuro-Ocular Eye Syndrome

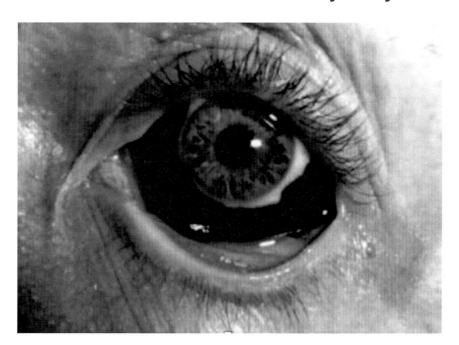

Information is creeping out through scientific circles that we may experience structural and functional changes to our eyes, which include optic-disc edema, globe flattening, choroidal folds, and hyperopic shifts or SANS for short.

It is thought that the ocular structural changes are triggered by the cephalad-fluid shift of people experiencing elevated $CO_2$ exposure, resistance exercise, radiation exposure, or elevated sodium intake. Because not all people develop SANS, some genetic, anatomical, or lifestyle related factors may incur greater susceptibility or protection to SANS.

Hypotheses to explain deficits in visual acuity and structural changes in the eye include elevated pressure in the vein and increased resistance in an outflow from the eye veins, increased intracranial pressure, the localized elevation of cerebrospinal fluid pressure within the sheath of the orbital optic nerve, and impaired drainage in the lymphatic system.

Many of the symptoms of SANS recover, although some structural changes are permanent or do not fully recover. It is currently unknown whether these structural changes will cause long-term decrements in visual acuity, visual fields, or have other functional consequences.

# SPE-like Radiation Effect on Gastrointestinal Tract Integrity

Numerous studies have been performed to evaluate the effects of SPE radiation on the immune system as a part of research on the acute risks of SPE radiation exposure. Studies related to immune system effects used mice exposed to doses of either gamma $\gamma$-ray or SPE- like proton radiation. The impacts of $\gamma$-ray and SPE-like proton radiation were comparable in these studies, and none of the observed effects described below were specific to proton or $\gamma$-ray radiation.

Your gastrointestinal (GI) tract contains over 1012 bacteria. These bacteria have many essential functions including carbohydrate fermentation and absorption, repression of pathogenic microbial growth, and continuous modulation of the gut and systemic immune system. They modulate everything from your mood to whether you will succumb to a virus. A critical function of the GI tract is the containment of commensal (friendly) bacteria, which involves the control of bacteria and bacterial product passage across the GI mucosa, known as bacterial translocation. This function can be disturbed in many different diseases. In one mouse study, gut changes began in as little as one-day post-exposure, causing a cascade of inflammatory, gut permeability, and activating the innate immune system-which when triggered can consume itself, much like Ouroboros, the snake eating its own tail. The innate system also has memory, so it is possible that because mankind has survived past events such as these, his or her cells remember these catastrophic events. For example, the fish in this article ran for cover before an earthquake! hit

Changes in gravity, radiation, hind leg suspension (HS) have been shown to cause a breakdown in the containment of Gram-negative bacterial products, as measured by circulating LPS. Stop the press. In the studies, I examined many referred to Hind-Leg Suspension. It is defined as A technique for limiting use, activity, or movement by immobilizing or restraining animals by suspending from hindlimbs or tails. This immobilization is used to simulate some effects of reduced gravity and study weightlessness physiology. It caught my attention because my old dog got hemangiosarcoma last fall. The first symptom that I noticed was the loss of his hind legs. I networked with many other dog owners whose dogs also had failed hind legs. Then I began to hear about people with leg problems with cancer. It just makes one think. I do not know the answer as yet, but there are more dots below.

I mention this for several reasons. Some gram-negative bacteria thrive in a vegetarian environment, and consequently, there is an uptick in these tenacious bacteria. Secondly, when I had a gram-negative bacterial infection and went through the airport scanner, the TSA interrogated me about what they saw on their screens. This is before I was symptomatic. Just letting you know, there are no more secrets.

Bacterial translocation can occur, which is when these bacteria penetrate the gut wall and go systemic. LBP was increased after treatment with proton radiation and was increased further when these stressors were combined.

These results demonstrate that circulating LPS, resulting from exposure to SPE-like radiation, led to a systemic response. It has been concluded from these studies that there is a synergistic effect when hindlimb-suspended mice are additionally exposed to SPE-like radiation.

These studies indicate that SPE-like radiation and hindlimb suspension induced breaks in the GI (gut) epithelial barrier and suggest that the increased frequency of interruptions could be responsible mechanistically for the increase in translocation of bacterial products into a system infection leading to sepsis and death.

# Risk of Cancer from Radiation

*Goodbye, my best friend. Hemangiosarcoma took your life, but you are always in my heart*

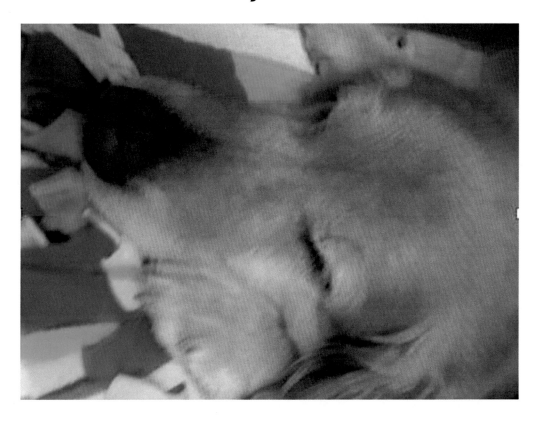

Everyone trembles at the dreaded word cancer. In the next few years, cancer is going to skyrocket due to the cosmic and nuclear superstorm. Other environmental factors, such as chemicals and synthetic biology, will also play a part. This is going to impact you, your loved ones, your friends, and even your pets/animals. NASA is predicting that there is "a possibility for increased cancer morbidity or mortality our lifetime." The agency is utilizing findings from the 2017 Potomac Institute report entitled "Projection of U.S. Cancer Mortality and Incidence Rates," to guide risk estimates and future research efforts.

From NASA: As there are distinct mechanisms of cancer induction across and within significant tissue sites, uncertainty reduction, requires tissue-specific risk estimates. NASA's Specialized Center of Research (NSCOR) is tasked with focusing on the critical sections of lung, breast, and colon; the blood system (leukemia's), liver, and brain for cancer. Understanding differences in radiation sensitivity based on genetic and epigenetic factors aid the development of tissue-specific cancer models, identification of biomarkers of both risk and early disease detection, and the identification of medical countermeasures that rely on advances current cancer research.

The cancer rate is the critical quantity in the evaluation, representing the probability of observing cancer at a given age and years since exposure. The life-span study of the Japanese survivors of the atomic bomb is the primary source for gamma-ray data. More recently, however, a meta-analysis of data for several tissue types from patients exposed to radiation or reactor workers has become available. These newer data will be used to compare with the Japanese data. Other assumptions in the model are made regarding the transfer of risk across populations, the use of average rates for the U.S. population, age, and age-after exposure dependence of risk on radiation quality and dose rate, etc.

Systems biology models provide a framework to integrate mechanistic studies of cancer risk across multiple levels of understanding (molecular, cellular, and tissue). Dosimetry in animal studies determined that simulated SPE radiation doses to the external organs (e.g., skin, eyes) are very high, while the doses to internal organs (e.g., spinal cord, bone marrow) are quite low. Animal tests indicate that the neutrophil count did not show a meaningful recovery by 3 months after exposure and that might the victim might be less capable of repairing DNA damage caused by the proton radiation exposure than the DNA damage caused by the electron radiation at similar or higher doses.

It has been pointed out in numerous current, and older reviews of space radiation carcinogenesis studies that space radiation-induced malignancies are dependent on the species, as well as the strain of the species used, and that a significant task in this field of research will involve determinations about the appropriate methods to use for extrapolation of the space radiation-induced cancer risks from experimental animal studies to humans.

One example of the differences observed in space radiation-induced cancer studies concerns the development of liver cell cancer. While exposure to space radiation(s) has indicated a very high incidence of liver cell cancer in one mouse strain, in other experiments on space radiation, induced carcinogenesis using a different strain of mice at a dose of 0.5 Gy from 56Fe ions or 3 Gy from protons. That later study showed had no effects on the development of hepatocellular carcinoma.

There are some intriguing recent results in the radiation carcinogenesis field of research. Ding et al. have indicated that there are distinct signatures (transcriptome profiles) in healthy human bronchial epithelial cells exposed to $\gamma$-rays and different HZE particles. If this effect can be confirmed, it may give rise to studies in which the causative agent can be identified in human malignancies that could have been caused by radiation exposure. While the mechanism(s) involved in space radiation-induced carcinogenesis are still unknown, there is evidence that space radiation-induced oxidative stress is closely associated with carcinogenesis. It has been reported that space radiation causes persistent oxidative stress in mouse intestine, which is likely to be related to intestinal tumorigenesis.

# Solutions and Countermeasure

Natural compounds or nutraceuticals with human health benefits are understandably attractive for use as radiation countermeasures because these compounds are found in our diets and are generally considered safe for clinical use as preventive or therapeutic agents. Nutraceuticals usually are thought to be more appropriate for medicinal use than "unnatural" synthetic analogs because nutraceuticals are well tolerated and have negligible toxicity, perhaps even when consumed in large quantities.

Vitamins are vital nutrients with diverse biochemical functions that are essential for maintaining health critical during stressful situations such as a nuclear or cosmic superstorm with all their compounding factors.

A "Countermeasure" is a specific protocol that is developed and validated to prevent or reduce the likelihood or consequence of a risk. Countermeasures may be medical, physical, or operational, such as a pharmaceutical or nutritional supplement, prototype hardware or software, or specific exercise routines.

Antioxidant supplementation, preferably from a food source, can aid in increasing the protection against cosmic radiation in persons. The type and the dose of the antioxidants must be adjusted according to age, sex, time spent at high altitudes and conditions related to the variations of the magnetosphere intensity, and solar activity. A healthy diet helps in the immunity processes. Oral administration of antioxidants before and during waves of cosmic rays can reduce radiation-induced oxidative stress.

Dog and cat owners: Please note that initially, I was going to extend this book to include protection for dogs and cats. The radioactive wave threat is underway, and I felt an urgency to get this material to you so that you have time to secure necessary items before they become unavailable at any price. Before giving any supplements to your dog or cat for radioactive protection, please conduct an internet search to see if it is safe or toxic for your pet.

Most of you are on a budget that is getting squeezed tighter by the day. What are health professionals and research recommendations for the essentials?

- **Vitamin C**

- **N acetylcysteine (NAC)**

- **L-selenomethionine is known as selenium- BEFORE whole-body irradiation can protect against oxidative damage**

- **Glutathione- especially useful for your liver, the detox organ in your body**

- **Lipoic acid**

- **Vitamin E- protect cells from the damaging effects of free radicals cause cancer**

- **Dried Prunes-powdered or dried fruit, not ray plums, dried have high protections due to concentration**

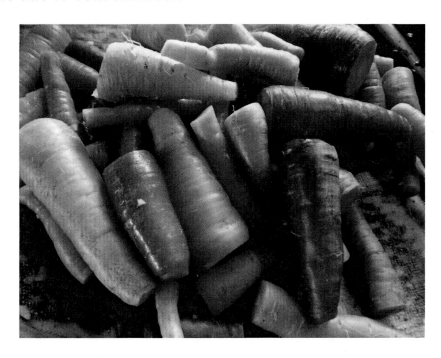

**Carrots, a great source of Vitamin A**

**If I was forced to choose two, I would select Vitamin C and Vitamin E. If I had some discretionary funds, I would include Vitamin A taken BEFORE whole-body irradiation can protect against the oxidative damage, melatonin, and fruit extracts which ameliorate deficits in behavior and signaling irradiated with 56 Fe ions. These are being effectively used in space travel to combat radiation.**

Flavonoid glycosides from Ginkgo biloba, myricetin, and quercetin have been postulated to improve cerebral metabolism, protect the brain against hypoxic damage (low oxygen) and scavenge free radicals.

Vitamin E and selenium, when used together synergistically, reduce 50% of chromosomal DNA abnormalities and oxidative stress when exposed to 2Gy of 6-Mv- x-rays radiation, with no side effects.

# Pharmaceutical Interventions

The following is a summary of the pharmaceutical interventions for radiation according to the NASA Human Research Program Integrated Research Plan, Human Research Program, published in March 2019:

Current medical treatment for acute radiation syndrome routinely includes supportive care:

• Antibiotics (quinolones and other agents),

• Cytokine therapy,

• Antiemetic agents (Reduce vomiting)

• Analgesic agents (pain relief)

Other agents can also be used for the effects of acute radiation syndrome:

• Antihistamines,

• Anti-inflammatory

• Radioprotectors

Several FDA approved anti-emetic drugs, such as Kytril (granisetron), Zofran (Ondansetron), Decadron® (dexamethasone tablets) and Emend (Aprepitant) are known to prevent or alleviate nausea and vomiting in patients or animals exposed to radiation or chemotherapeutic agents.

Amifostine significantly reduces the side effects of radiation but has harsh side effects:

• Protect against DNA damage in cisplatin-treated murine peripheral leukocytes,

- Reduce changes in nucleolar morphology

- Protect against disruption of taste

- Protect against small intestinal mucositis,

- Inhibit tumor formation

PrC-210 is a new aminothiol that has shown no detectable nausea/vomiting or hypotension side effects in animal models, in contrast to the strong side effects of the current aminothiol, amifostine. This compound shows promise as a new aminothiol radioprotector.

Interferon mitigates acute radiation effects on the immune system and also an active Hexose correlated compound, which activates immune function and enhances resistance to infection.

Space radiation cancer is prevented/mitigated by chemo-preventive agents, protease inhibitors, and HIV enzyme.

## OTC-Cimetidine

Cimetidine (brand name Tagamet-OTC) is an antagonist of histamine type II receptors, basically, an antihistamine that works on a different pathway than say Benedryl.

- Radioprotective

- Inhibits apoptosis Programmed cell death

- Protects the Lymph system

- Protects immature stem cells

- Useful for both LET low and high radiation

- Protects against whole-body gamma radiation

Radioprotective

Vitamins & Supplements

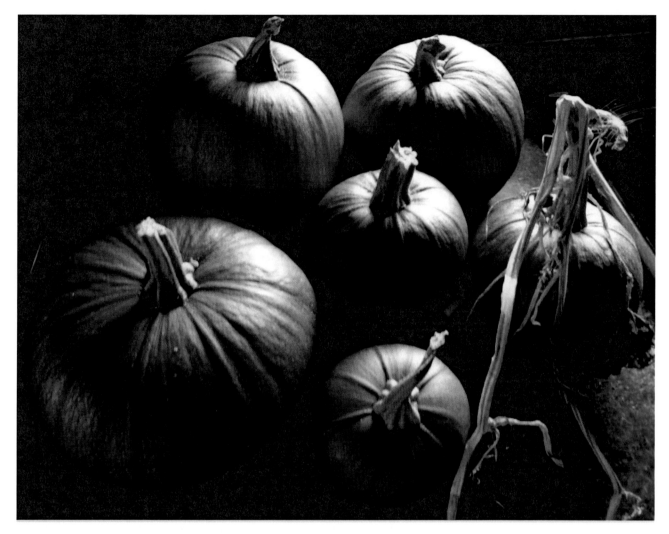

Vitamin A

**Pumpkins are a joy to grow. Yes! You can grow them in your windowsill**

**Vitamin A or beta carotene vitamin. Vitamin A retinol and dehydroretinol found in animal foods, primarily the liver and milk fat, can be toxic. It used to be called the miracle vitamin because of its effect on the immune system.**

**• Radioprotective**

**• Manufactures antibodies,**

**• Maintains and protects mucous membranes and**

**• Protects the thymus gland, the master gland of the immune system.**

• Helps guard against tumor formation and cancer,

• Reverses the aging process of the skin caused by ultraviolet light, which includes cosmic rays

DUAL Purpose: Vitamin A is involved with numerous bodily processes, including vision, growth, bone and tooth development, skin, healthy mucosa, and protection against cancer. They also contain antioxidants that protect the heart and arteries. I personally find that Vitamin A supplementation during the first 5 days of any signs of infection often eliminates or reduces a viral or bacterial infection. Anti Aging, may help hyperthyroidism, improves night vision.

Deficiency includes vision disorders, dry skin, and fetal development disorders.

Processing: 15-35% of Vitamin A is lost in cooking. Sunlight, ultraviolet light, destroys vitamin A. Freezing does not impact Vitamin A.

Fact-Checker: Carrots and apricots have the highest plant-based Vitamin A. Beef liver and butter have the highest animal-based Vitamin A.

Food availability: Provitamin A includes carotenes and beta-carotenes found in orange vegetables, carrots, peppers, and some dark greens such as spinach, and present no risk of toxicity.

Lima beans, potatoes, yams, sweet potatoes, asparagus, tomatoes, onions and spinach, fruits (mango, grapes, avocado, pears, oranges, plus the white under the peel and pulps, apples plus seeds and skin, strawberries), all unsprouted seeds (especially sunflower, sesame, and pumpkin), all nuts (especially almonds and cashews), leafy green vegetables, carob and teas from fruit blossoms and leaves (peach flowers, strawberry leaves, cherry flowers, apple blossoms), and all grasses, such as wheat and barley. The vitamin A analog, abscisic acid, is found in large amounts in the grasses, seeds, nuts, legumes, mature leaves and fruits listed above and in the apricot pit. The body makes abscisic acid inside your body from raw carrot juice and raw liver.

Let's go wild!

Plantain   Wild Strawberries   Dandelion   Water Cress

Chickweed   Elderberry Flower   Lambs Quarters Purslane

**Nettles   Rose Hips    Calendula**

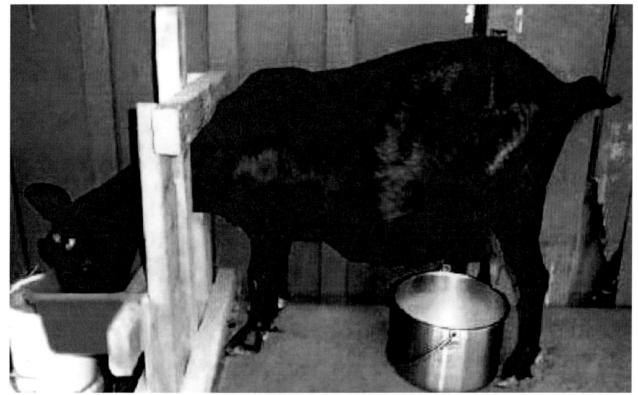

Vitamin B 12

**What is it? Cyanocobalamin or Methylcobalamin**

**Where is it found? Higher animals do not produce this vitamin, but they store it in their liver. Milk and eggs and fish contain B12. Specific yeasts during fermentation can produce B12.**

**What is its function? B12 is necessary for cell division, the formation of red blood cells, and the formation of myelin, the fiber that protects the nerves.**

**• Radioprotective**

**SYNERGY effect: Vitamin B12 and folic acid supplementation in rats may defend against radiation-induced oxidative stress and leukopenia.**

**Let's go wild!**

- **Wild Amaranth**

- **Wild Sea Buckthorn**

**Deficiency symptoms: Anemia and nervous disorders. I can attest that being low in B12 can impact cognition and energy also.**

**When to increase it: If you are a vegetarian.**

**Processing: Cooking destroys 30% of B12, pasteurization of milk about 10%**

**Fact checker: Beer and white bread are the highest sources of plant-based B12 while animal-based B12 is found in animal liver, caviar, fish, and eggs.**

## Bee Pollen

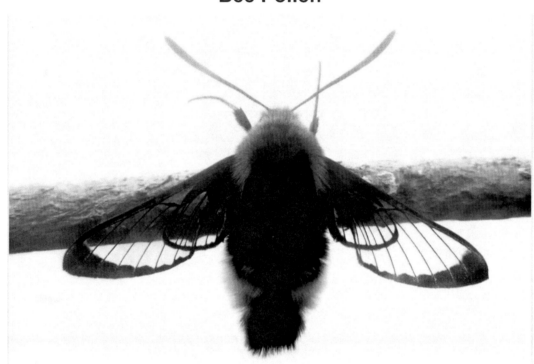

*If you do not have 25 species of pollinators in your garden, there is something wrong. Yes, for a higher yield, I do play pollinator daily.*

**Pollen is an excellent food containing all essential amino acids, vitamins A, D, E, K, C, bioflavonoids, B-complex (especially pantothenic acid and B3), and 27 minerals.**

- **Radioprotective for immature stem cells**

• Research has proven pollen to be beneficial in treating several diseases.

• Dr. Emil Chauvin (French Academy of Science) discovered bee pollen helped treat anemia (increases red blood cells and hemoglobin),

• Chronic prostatitis, Constipation, Flatulence, Colon infections, especially diarrhea.

• In one study, 25 women with inoperative uterine cancer. All received radiotherapy. The 15 who took 20 grams of bee pollen three times a day tolerated the radiation much better than the 10 who took no bee pollen.

Propolis and lycopene have radioprotective properties against UVA radiation 01, 2006

Substances: Bee Propolis, Diseases: Photo dermatosis, Sunburn, Pharmacological Actions : Radioprotective

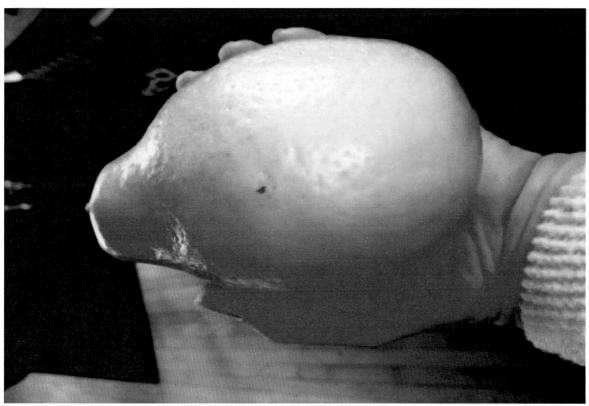

Vitamin C

*I grew this monster lemon in my windowsill in -50 Fahrenheit. The tree had 100 lemons in this size. This is a Meyer Lemon.*

**What is it? Ascorbic acid.**

**Where is it found? Plants and most animals can synthesize it from glucose, but humans cannot, nor can they store it. It must be taken daily!**

**According to Valko et al., The role of vitamin C supplementation:**

**• Reduces of DNA damages, in the protein and the lipid oxidation -think of that as body rust.**

**• Directly interacts with hydroxyl (HO·) resulted during oxidative stress and formed less toxic free radicals**

**• Vitamin C decreases upon exposure to radiation in these organs: liver, brain, and spleen. That is why supplementation with this antioxidant helps in protection against oxidative stress produced by ionizing radiation.**

**SYNERGY Effect: Vitamin C + bioflavonoid & rutin.**

**Dosage: A protective dose of between 500mg and 2,000 mg can counteract toxins and radiation.**

**What is its function?**

**• It is an antioxidant that neutralizes free radicals, which cause cellular aging, DNA deterioration, and cancer.**

**• It is an antitoxin that neutralizes a variety of toxins, including those found in cured meat.**

**• It strengthens the immune system against infection.**

**• Contributes to collagen formation and is necessary for wound healing.**

**• It improves bones and teeth.**

**• Strengthens capillary and arterial walls.**

• Facilitates absorption of nonheme iron.

Deficiency symptoms: Fatigue, poor wound healing, bleeding, scurvy

When to increase it: Nicotine addiction, stress, infection, wound, burns

Processing: Vitamin C is the most sensitive of all vitamins. Heat, light, dehydration destroys 75% of this Vitamin C.

Fact checker: Beef liver, oyster, trout are the highest animal-based source of Vitamin C, while Red Sweet Peppers, Guava, and Black currants are the highest plant-based Vitamin C sources. Rose hips can be used for high vitamin C but they must be used fresh, or they lose their Vitamin C.

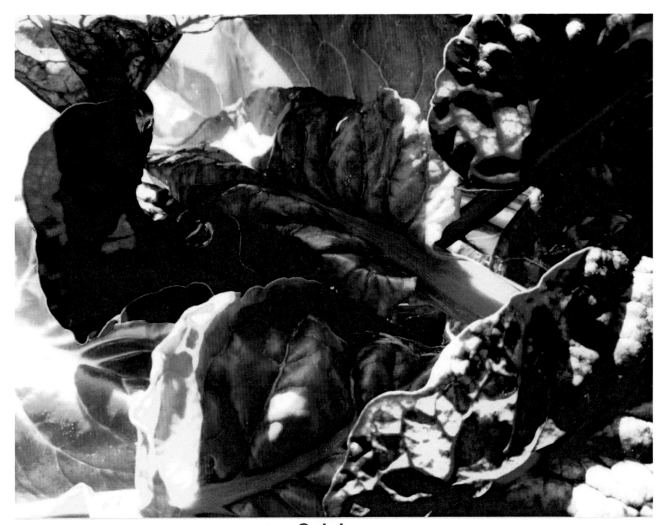
Calcium

*Bright Lights Swiss Chard greens a delicious summer treat and make a wonderful Swiss Chard and Goat Cheese Galette (below)*

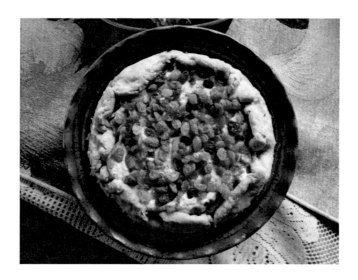

**What is it? A mineral**

Radiation, because of its structure, tricks the body into up taking radioisotopes instead of calcium, much to the detriment of the biological life form. This is true in humans, animals, and plants.

• Calcium, according to The New England Journal of Medicine, may prevent precancerous cells from becoming cancerous.

• Protects against Strontium 90 (similar in structure to calcium) and other radioisotopes.

**What is its function?**

Calcium is involved in bone and teeth formation, muscular contraction, nerve impulse transmission, and blood coagulation.

Only 20-30% of the calcium in food is absorbed by the intestines.

Vitamin D, dietary protein, and milk facilitate calcium absorption.

Phosphorous (rich in meat and fish), phytate in bran, oxalates such as rhubarb, spinach, leafy greens can inhibit calcium absorption.

Where is it found? Milk, dairy sesame, blackstrap molasses, beans, cabbage, and oranges.

Let's go wild!

Plaintain   Lambs quarters   Onions  Gromwell

Nettle    Lungwort   Chickweed   Purslane

Red Clover

Deficiency symptoms: Rickett's, osteoporosis

When to increase it: Young, pregnancy, nursing

Processing: Minimal loss of calcium occurs during cooking.

Fact checker: Dairy products, sardines, and eggs are high in calcium while sesame, molasses, beans, and chard are high plant-based calcium sources.

## CBD Oil

CBD stands for cannabidiol. It is the second most prevalent of the active ingredients of cannabis (marijuana). While CBD is an essential component of medical marijuana, it is derived directly from the hemp plant, which is a cousin of the marijuana plant. While CBD is a component of marijuana (one of the hundreds), by itself, it does not cause a "high." According to a report from the World Health Organization, "In humans, CBD exhibits no effects indicative of any abuse or dependence potential.... To date, there is no evidence of public health-related problems associated with the use of pure CBD."

Is cannabidiol legal?

CBD is readily obtainable in most parts of the United States, though its exact legal status is in flux. All 50 states have laws legalizing CBD with varying degrees of restriction, and while the federal government still considers CBD in the same class as marijuana, it doesn't habitually enforce against it. CBD has been shown to improve cellular communication and healthy cellular proliferation, two things ionizing radiation disrupt.

High-grade glioma is one of the most aggressive cancers in adult humans, and long-term survival rates are meager as standard treatments for glioma remain largely unsuccessful. Cannabinoids have been shown to specifically inhibit glioma growth as well as neutralize oncogenic processes such as angiogenesis.

CBD oil provides radio-protective qualities:

• Improve brain and liver function

• An anti-inflammatory

• Reduces Pain

• Reduces nausea and vomiting

• Reduces anxiety

• Reduce microbial contamination

• Antitumor activity

My source for CBS oil is The Source.

# Chlorophyll

**Chlorophyll closely resembles human blood. It used to cleanse, detoxify, purify, and heal many conditions.**

• **Radioprotective**

• **Retards bacterial growth,**

• **Detoxifies heavy metals from the body,**

• **Increases wound healing,**

• **Detoxifies the liver and other organs,**

• **Deodorizes the body,**

• **Removes putrefactive bacteria from the colon,**

• **Aids healing of 11 types of skin diseases,**

• **Relieves ulcers, gastritis, pancreatitis, and other inflammatory conditions,**

• **Helps heal gum diseases**

• **Inhibits metabolic activation of many carcinogens**

**Many studies have reported the protective effects of chlorophyll on irradiated animals. There are pure chlorophyll supplements available if you don't like to eat grass or algae. Chlorophyll-containing foods: barley grass and chlorella.**

# Chlorella

**Chlorella is a green freshwater micro-alga which has even more chlorophyll than barley (wheat) grass plus 55-65% protein with 19 amino acids, including all the essential ones. It's an excellent source of beta-carotene, vitamins B-l, B-2, B-3, B-6, B-12, pantothenic acid, folic acid, biotin, PABA, inositol and vitamin C. Vitamin B-12 is especially important for vegetarians who may be deficient in this vitamin. Chlorella has more B-12 than the liver. It also contains essential minerals - iron, phosphorus, magnesium, calcium, zinc, potassium, sulfur, iodine and trace**

amounts of manganese, sodium and chlorine. Chlorella comes in a small pill form, which may be more palatable to some people.

## CoQ 10

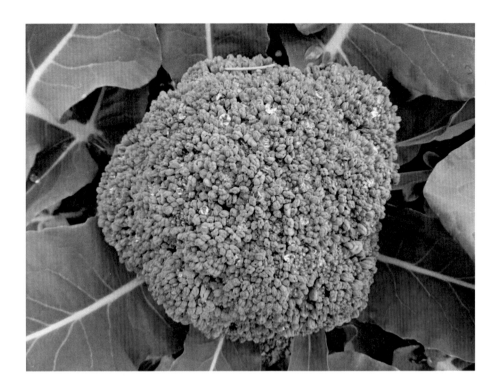

*It is getting more challenging to grow due to climatic extremes. It can bolt in a day.*

Coenzyme Q10 is an essential chemical that the body produces naturally. A deficiency of this chemical can have adverse effects, and coenzyme Q10 supplements may offer health benefits. Also called: Ubiquinol. This coenzyme decreases with age. For maximum benefit, it is recommended to supplement it.

• CoQ10 naturally decreases with age, and so supplementation is critical.

• Radioprotective

• Chemical protective

• Boosts immune system

• Retards aging

- Anti Inflammatory

- Reduces oxidative stress

- Reduces apoptosis (programmed cell death)

- Reduces cancer

Sufferers of heart problems, high blood pressure, angina, and obesity often find this substance to help manage symptoms.

Food availability: Cabbage, Broccoli, Oysters, Beef liver, Avocados, Oranges

# DHEA

DHEA The most dominant hormone in the body.

- DHEA is considered the "Fountain of Youth" hormone because it can help extend life DHEA helps counteract the adverse effects of stress,

- Boosts the immune system,

- Regulates blood cholesterol

- It lowers blood pressure.

- It rebalances the hormones in the body, especially during menopause,

- Inhibits the growth of cancer

- Reduces fat

- Reduces osteoporosis associated with irradiation

- Anti-Aging

Food availability: wild yams

# Vitamin E

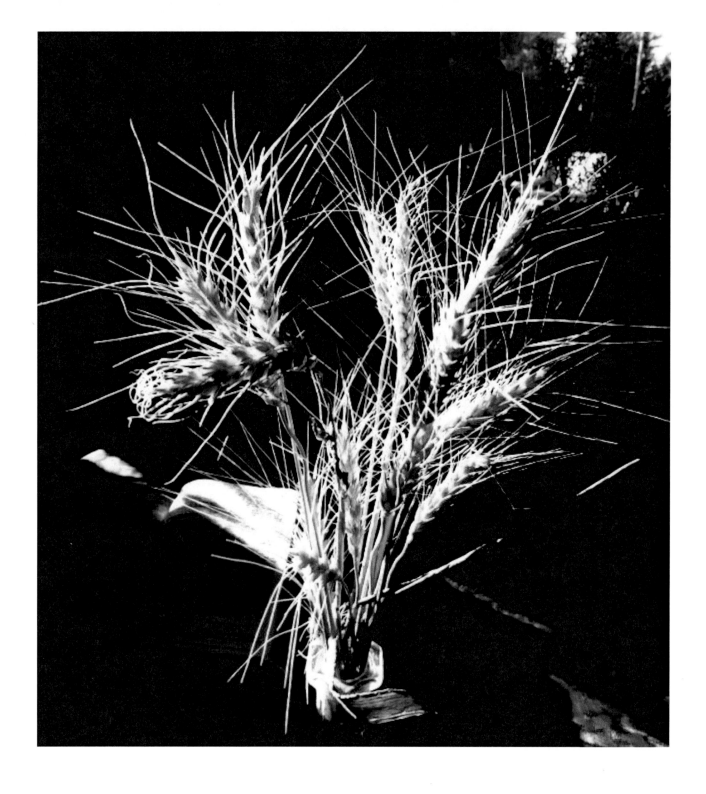

*This is what happens why you mulch with a wheat straw? Lovely and eatable wheat throughout your garden.*

What is it? Vitamin E was first identified in the 1930s as a dietary ingredient essential for the maintenance of fertility and consequently derived its name from the Greek words "tokos" and "pherein" that together signify the "bearing of offspring." Tocopherols have the potential to protect healthy cells from radiation-induced mutations.

Is a generic term for all biologically active compounds of tocopherols and tocotrienols which are fat-soluble nutrients that are:

• Radioprotective

• Anti-Cancer

• Antioxidant,

• Neuroprotective, and

• Anti-inflammatory properties

• Anti-tumor mechanism

• Protects intestinal (gut mucosa) from whole-body gamma radiation if administered

Where is it found? It is located in grain germ, particularly wheat, sunflower seeds, nuts, olives, avocado.

What is its function?

• Vitamin E protects the integrity of the cells and prolongs their life span.

• It is an antioxidant that prevents oxidation of vegetable oils.

• Neutralizes harmful free radicals from chemical contamination and body activity within cell walls.

• Protective action against cancer and arteriosclerosis (hardening of the arteries)

• Involved in the formation of germinal cells (reproduction).

Vitamin E is known to have antioxidant properties capable of scavenging free radicals, which have critical roles in radiation injuries. Tocopherols and tocotrienols, vitamin E analogs, are together known as tocols, have shown promise as radioprotectors.

**Important to know:** There is more than one type of Vitamin E. Tocotrienols have shown superior antioxidant activity to tocopherols, with one report documenting tocotrienols having 1600 times' higher antioxidant activity than α-tocopherol.

**SYNERGY Effect:** Administration of vitamins E and C, to block the DNA damage, lipid peroxidation, and proteins oxidation and to inhibit the oxidative stress in testicular tissue.

**Dosage:** Vitamin E supplementation with doses lower than 200 IU/day is considered beneficial and protects the cell membranes against lipid peroxidation induced by radiation.

**FLEETING WINDOW OF OPPORTUNITY:** The window of radioprotection for α-tocopherol is about 24 h with circulating blood levels of α-tocopherol peaking at 24 h and at 4 h.

**When to administer:** 15 minutes before the irradiation and for 13 days after irradiation, also subcutaneous (under the skin) 24 h before radiation exposure has shown protective effects against ARS.

**Foods with Vitamin E:** Peanut, wheat, and soybeans have more tocopherols than tocotrienols, whereas oats, barley, palm oil, and rice bran oil have more tocotrienols.

| Sources | Tocopherol (milligram/1000 grams) | | | | | Tocotrienol (milligram/1000 grams) | | | | |
|---|---|---|---|---|---|---|---|---|---|---|
| | Alpha | Beta | Gamma | Delta | Total | Alpha | Beta | Gamma | Delta | Total |
| Palm oil | 152 | | | | 152 | 205 | | 439 | 94 | 738 |
| Rice barn | 324 | 18 | 53 | | 395 | 116 | | 349 | | 465 |
| Barley | 350 | 50 | 50 | | 450 | 670 | 120 | 120 | | 910 |
| Oat | 180 | 20 | 50 | 50 | 300 | 180 | | 30 | | 210 |
| Coconut oil | 5 | | | 6 | 11 | 5 | 1 | 19 | | 25 |
| Wheat germ | 1179 | 398 | 493 | 118 | 2188 | 24 | 165 | | | 189 |
| Palm kernel oil | 13 | | | | 13 | 21 | | | | 21 |
| Soya bean oil | 101 | | 593 | 264 | 958 | | | | | 0 |
| Sunflower oil | 387 | | 387 | | 774 | | | | | 0 |
| Peanut oil | 130 | | 216 | 21 | 367 | | | | | 0 |
| Cocoa butter | 11 | | 170 | 17 | 198 | 2 | | | | 2 |
| Olive oil | 51 | | | | 51 | | | | | 0 |

The vitamin E derivatives that have shown significant activity after acute exposure to ionizing radiation and have the potential to be further developed as radiation countermeasures.

## Tocopherols (Vitamin E)

(1) Alpha-Tocopherol. The radioprotective properties of tocopherols have been demonstrated in several recent reports. In one such study, subcutaneous administration of $\alpha$-tocopherol (100 IU/kg body weight) either 1 h before or 15 min after $\gamma$-irradiation significantly increased the 30-day survival of mice. Higher subcutaneous doses of $\alpha$-tocopherol (400 IU/kg body weight) enhanced the survival of irradiated mice when given 24 h before $\gamma$-irradiation.

NOTATION: Oral administration of $\alpha$-tocopherol significantly reduced the frequency of micronuclei formation and chromosomal aberrations in the bone marrow cells of mice exposed to 1 Gy of radiation.

HOW IT WORKS: When exposed to gamma-irradiation followed immediately by the administration of $\alpha$-tocopherol results in a surge in the number of new immature stem cells (that can become any type of cell) in the spleen suggesting that α-tocopherol also stimulates recovery or repair processes

One study indicated that the mitigative radio effects of α-tocopherol may result from its ability to enhance cell-mediated immunity.

 (2Alpha-Tocopherol-MonoglucosideAlpha-tocopherol-monoglucoside or αTMG is a water-soluble derivative of α-tocopherol. Because αTMG is soluble in water, it is a better candidate than other forms of vitamin E for development as a radiation countermeasure agent.

**Experiments:**

• Demonstrate that oral administration of αTMG at doses of up to 7 g/Kg body weight was nontoxic in a mouse model, and protected mice from weight loss and death and shifted lethal death dosage from 6 Gy to 6.72 Gy.

• When given before a dose of 2 Gy of radiation, αTMG reduced the radiation-induced mortality among embryos of pregnant mice by 75%.

• Protected against both radiation-induced chromosomal damage and

• Radiation-induced formation of thymine glycol.

• αTMG protects the immature stem cell recovery of irradiated mice

• Mitigate radiation-induced bone marrow damage

• Suggests that αTMG can protect DNA

(3) Gamma-Tocopherol-N, N-Dimethylglycine Ester. Gamma-tocopherol-N, N-dimethylglycine ester (GTDMG) is a water-soluble derivative of tocopherol and a prodrug of γ-tocopherol

A recent evaluation of the protective effects of GTDMG in mice showed that it significantly enhanced 30-day survival when given 30 min before or just after irradiation.

**Dosage:**

• Giving GTDMG at 100 mg/Kg body weight intraperitoneally to mice 30 min before TBI with 7.5 Gy significantly protected the bone marrow and increased the survival rate of the mice by 70%.

• Giving the same concentration immediately after irradiation led to survival rates of about 98%, with a DRF of 1.25, and even giving GTDMG at 24 h after irradiation showed significant mitigation effects.

(4) Alpha-Tocopherol Succinate. Alpha-tocopherol succinate, the hemisuccinate ester derivative of α-tocopherol, is:

• Promising anti-tumor agent

• Protection against chromosomal damage

• Protection against radiation-induced apoptosis and cytotoxicity

• Reduced DNA damage and apoptosis (cell death)

• Inhibits bacterial translocation from gut to the bloodstream, which is similar to the blood-brain barrier only in the stomach. Radiation allows bacteria to permeate through the gut wall.

• Reduces inflammation in gut tissues

• Preserves the intestinal barrier when exposed to radiation

  In mice, α-tocopherol succinate was protective against ARS in a dose-dependent manner; when administered 24 h before irradiation, it can protect mice from acute doses of γ-radiation with a DRF of 1.28. In fact, a single treatment of TS (400 mg/Kg body weight), given 24 hours before 60Co γ-radiation exposure, enhanced the survival rate of mice with gastrointestinal ARS by alleviating radiation-induced intestinal injuries and improving overall intestinal health.

Improvements in survival were achieved from transfusion of stem cell-enriched peripheral blood mononuclear cells from the α-tocopherol succinate-treated mice serves as a kind of "bridge" therapy until recovery of your innate immune system from radiation exposure.

For your physician only:

In terms of its effects on the hematopoietic system, α-tocopherol succinate has been found to reduce neutropenia, thrombocytopenia, and monocytopenia, but not to affect lymphocyte counts, in irradiated mice. To abolish the protective effect of α-tocopherol succinate against ARS.

Transfusion of whole blood or peripheral blood mononuclear cells allows irradiated mice to survive doses of radiation that typically elicit the GI syndrome

Dosage: optimal radioprotection noted when α-tocopherol succinate is given 24 h before TBI.

Potential advantages of using α-tocopherol succinate rather than G-CSF for cytokine therapy are its low cost and ease of storage and administration in a mass casualty situation.

(1) Gamma-Tocotrienol. Gamma-tocotrienol or γT3 has potent antioxidant properties as well as inhibiting HMG-CoA reductase, similar to statins.

It appears to be associated with an increase in various blood cells in the peripheral blood, suggesting faster stem cell recovery.

Dosage: Administered at doses of 100 mg/Kg body weight and 200 mg/Kg body weight at 24 h before 60Co radiation, γT3 protected mice from death after radiation doses as high as 11.5 Gy, with a DRF of 1.29.

For your physician only:

• γT3 effectively mobilizes hematopoietic progenitors in the peripheral blood, thereby enhancing its radioprotective action.

• Aside from its effects on cytokines and hematopoietic cells, γT3 also reduces radiation-induced oxidative stress within blood vessels, which was readily reversed by mevalonate.

• γT3 even reversed the decrease in tetrahydrobiopterin in the lungs induced by irradiation.

• Vitamin E as a strategy to reduce or reverse late radiation-induced cardiac, pulmonary, intestinal, skeletal, and dermal fibrosis

Advancement of γT3 as a radiation countermeasure for human use will require documentation of its pharmacokinetics, pharmacodynamics, and radioprotective efficacy in nonhuman primate models.

(2) Delta-Tocotrienol. Like γT3, delta-tocotrienol (δT3) also has potent antioxidant properties that can be exploited for radioprotection.

Dosage: Administered as a single subcutaneous dose 24 h before 60Co γ-irradiation, δT3 at 150 mg/Kg body weight, and at 300 mg/Kg body weight protected mice with respective DRFs of 1.19 and 1.27. Radioprotective efficacy has been documented from doses ranging from 18.75 mg/Kg body weight to 400 mg/Kg body weight. When administered 2 h after radiation, the DRF for 150 mg/Kg body weight of δT3 was observed to be 1.1.

It protects the bone marrow and stem cells radiation injury primarily by suppressing the radiation-induced microRNA-30 and other signaling pathways.

α-tocopherol succinate mobilizes immature stem cells to protect against exposure to a broad range of radiation doses but does not seem to mitigate radiation-induced effects when given after radiation exposure.

Despite these early indications of efficacy, further exploratory research is required to (a) develop biocompatible vehicles and formulations for improved bioavailability, (b) evaluate the safety and tolerability of different formulations, routes of administration, and dosing strategies, (c) decipher the mechanism of action at a molecular level, (d) extend efficacy studies to nonhuman primates, (e) investigate the synergistic effect of tocols with other radioprotectors, and (f) identify non-invasive biological markers of efficacy in humans to confirm delivery of an adequate dose.

Let's go wild!

• Watercress                    Purslane                    Sheep Sorrel

• Spirula              Rose Hips

Deficiency symptoms:

• Patients with vitamin E deficiency may show signs and symptoms of hyporeflexia that progress to ataxia, including limitations in upward gaze.

• Patients may present with profound muscle weakness and visual-field constriction.

• Patients with severe, prolonged vitamin E deficiency may develop complete blindness, cardiac arrhythmia, and dementia.

When to increase it: When consuming vegetable oils rich in polyunsaturated fats.

Processing:

Refined grains lose 80%

Roasted nuts lose: 80%

Frying in oil lost 32-75%

Preserves lost 41-65%

Fact checker: Flatfish, butter, and fresh eggs are the best source of Vitamin E for animal-based while plant-based Vitamin E can be found in wheat germ oil, sunflower oil, and all of your nuts, seeds, and oils.

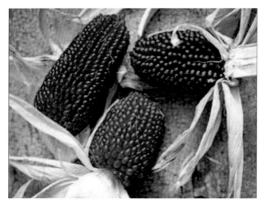
Ferulic Acid

*Heirloom Strawberry Popcorn is easy to grow and fun to eat*

What is it? Ferulic acid (4-hydroxy-3-methoxy cinnamic acid), a phenolic compound found in the cell wall of plants, is a potent free-radical scavenger and antioxidant. Concerning its hepatoprotective effect, ferulic acid has been shown to decrease the elevated serum levels of the liver marker enzymes AST, ALT, alkaline phosphatase (ALP), and gamma-glutamyl transferase (GGT) in rats subjected to ethanol-induced hepatotoxicity.

• **Radioprotective**

• **Antioxidant**

• **Ameliorates oxidative stress**

• **Protective against low dose radiation**

• **Protective against cosmic radiation**

• **Inhibits DNA damage after exposure to gamma radiation**

• **Initiatives cell repair processes**

• **The nuclear factor erythroid 2-related factor 2, Nrf2, is a transcription factor that regulates the expression of antioxidant proteins, playing an important key role in ROS scavenging, even in radiation exposure.**

**When: After exposure to ionizing radiation**

**DUAL use: Anti-Aging, beneficial in the prevention and/or treatment of various disorders linked to oxidative stress, such as Alzheimer's disease, diabetes, cancer, cardiovascular disease, and atherosclerosis (as reviewed in Zhao and Moghadasian139).**

**It's found naturally in the seeds of fruits like apples and oranges, as well as some vegetables, nuts, and grains, and fights the free-radical damage that contributes to aging. According to Angela Lamb, an assistant professor of dermatology at Mount Sinai Hospital in New York City, as long as you don't have susceptible skin or an allergy to ferulic acid, it's an excellent ingredient for slowing the hands of time.**

Ginkgo Gilboa

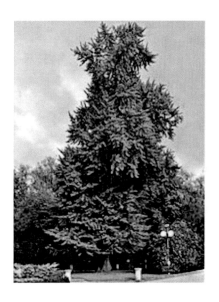

*Stately health*

Ginkgo biloba is an antioxidant-rich herb used to enhance brain health and treat a variety of conditions.

• Has been postulated to improve cerebral metabolism,

• Protect the brain against hypoxia (low oxygen) damage and

• Scavenge free radicals

DUAL USE: Check for other benefits

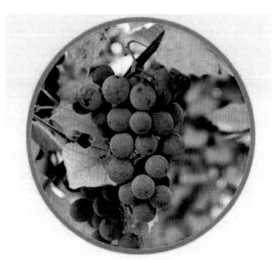

Grape Seed Extract

*Many grape varieties are hardy to -30. Grapes sweeten after frosts so do not pick too early*

The grape seed extract is an industrial derivative of grape seeds. It is rich in antioxidants and oligomeric pro-anthocyanidin complexes and has been linked to a wide range of possible health benefits.

One of the most potent antioxidants or free radical scavengers,

• GSE helps counteract stress,

• GSE counteracts pollution

• GSE counteracts radiation

DUAL USE for many health benefits

## Iodine

Iodine prevents DNA double-strand breaks induced by radio iodide-(131) I in thyroid cells. Mar 01, 2011, Substances: Iodine, Diseases: Radiation-Induced Illness: Radioiodine (Iodine-131), Pharmacological Actions: Radioprotective

## Lipoic Acid

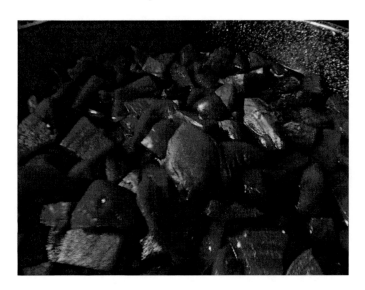

*Beets are an excellent supply for Lipoic Acid. I like mine, spicy pickled!*

Lipoic acid is a lipid and water-soluble compound, an antioxidant.

• Radioprotective

• **Lipoic acid can protect against oxidative stress produced by radiation**

• **Protects ovary and testicular cells**

• **Protects immature stem cells**

**SYNERGY effect: Protects cell membranes when it interacts with vitamin C and glutathione.**

**Dihydrolipoic acid (DHLA), the reduced form of lipoic acid, is a much more potent antioxidant, being able to regenerate other endogenous antioxidants from their radical way.**

**DUAL USE: For diabetes and nerve symptoms from diabetes, including burning, pain, and numbness in the legs and arms.**

## Lycopene

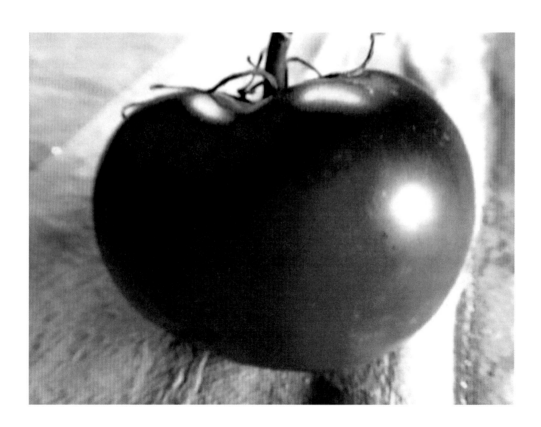

*Many heirloom varieties are beginning to bump up the Lycopene.  You will see it on seed labels, but not so much plant starts.  This is a stunning Indigo Apple, 6*

*ounces, with a rich tomato taste! Tomatoes do love lots of water to get the size. Watch for early and late blight.*

**Lycopene, an Nrf2 enhancer, is a carotenoid that gives some vegetables and fruits their red color. It is found in tomatoes, carrots, watermelon, and papayas.**

**You will discover many new heirloom varieties breeding in high lycopene into various fruits and vegetables. The seed or plant starts will notify you that this species is high in lycopene. I have been experimenting with multiple varieties, and I am enjoying the flavor and nutrient density of these lycopene enhanced varieties.**

**• Radioprotective**

**• Strong antioxidant**

**• Protects lymphocytes BEFORE radiation**

**DUAL USE: It can be used for many health conditions.**

Lycopene protects against gamma-radiation induced DNA damage, lipid peroxidation, and oxidative stress in rat hepatocytes in vitro. Apr 01, 2007

**Substances: Carotenoids, Lycopene, Diseases: DNA damage, Radiation-Induced Illness, Pharmacological Actions: Antioxidants, Hepatoprotective, Radioprotective**

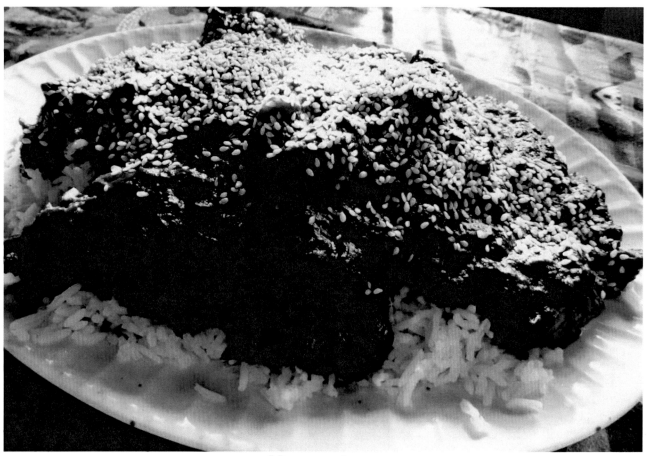

Magnesium

*Mole has lots of sesame seeds, nuts, and chocolate! When you grow your own Mole peppers and all the ingredients, it is much more flavorful, and you can customize for your personal taste sensation! In this way, you save seed diversity and indigenous recipes.*

**What is it? A mineral.**

**• Radioprotective (serine-magnesium sulfate mixture as a new, non-toxic, potent and efficient radioprotective agent)**

**Where is it found? Wheat bran is the richest product in magnesium. It contains 20 times more than in milk or meat. But due to the phytates, very little is absorbed. Look to legumes, sesame, and oil-bearing nuts also. 30-50% is absorbed from foods.**

**What is its function?**

Magnesium is involved in the formation of bones and teeth, serves as a catalyst in energy production reactions within the cells, facilitates the transmission of nerve impulses, is concerned with muscle relaxation, as opposed to calcium, which promotes muscle contractions.

Facilitates absorption of food proteins, lactose from milk, and Vitamin D.

It inhibits excess calcium and phosphorous. Excellent pain killer.

DUAL USE: Leg cramps, migraine headaches, muscle spasms, constipation, and especially to lower blood pressure in patients with hypertension.

**Let's go wild!**

• Onion

• Cabbage

• Apple

• Hickory Bark

• Purslane

• Milk

• Red Clover

Deficiency symptoms: Generalized muscle spasms.

When to increase it: Alcoholism, diarrhea, kidney disorders

Processing: Very little is lost in processing.

**Food availability:** Dairy, fish, shellfish, and beef are good sources of magnesium while bran, seeds and nuts, molasses fruit, and even real chocolate syrup provides plant-based magnesium.

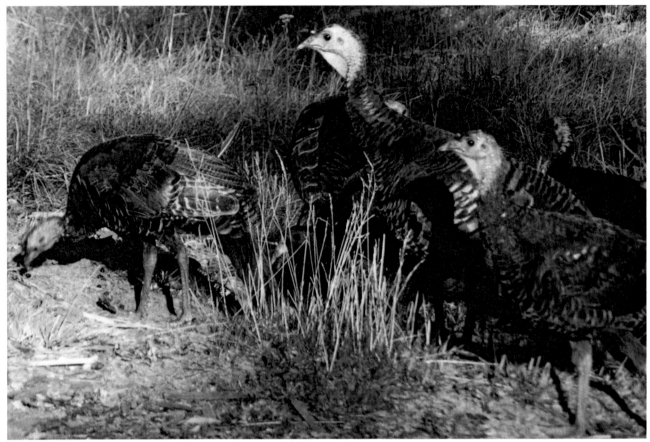

Melatonin

*Rush hour in the Rockies*

Melatonin is a hormone found naturally in the body. Melatonin used as medicine is usually made synthetically in a laboratory.

• **Radioprotective**

• **Antioxidant**

• **Protects against oxidative stress**

• **May protect the eye lens from to gamma-radiation**

- Protection against cataract development

- Cancer inhibiting hormone

- Protects the pineal gland from electric field exposure

DUAL USE: Pineal gland, sleep cycle (circadian), insomnia, fertility, and immune system, prevents jet lag, anti-aging, anti-inflammatory, neuroprotective, control of cardiovascular disease, diabetes, obesity, regulates moods, control body temperature.

New research in periodontology.

Sources of melatonin in food:

- Lamb

- Beef

- Pork

- Salmon

- Chicken/turkey

# Melatonin has radiosensitizing properties in leukemia cells and radioprotective properties in normal cells. Sep 01, 2009

Substances: Melatonin

Diseases: Acute T cell Leukemia's

Pharmacological Actions: Apoptotic, Bcl-2 protein down-regulation, Radioprotective, Radiosensitizer, Tumor Suppressor Protein p53 Upregulation

# Myricetin

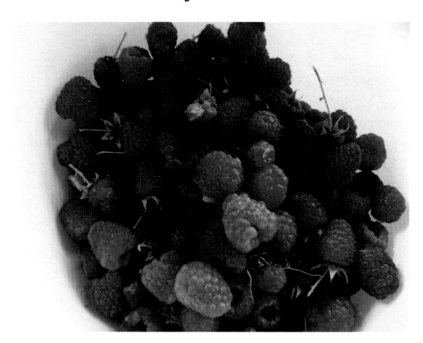

*Think flavor here!  I am getting bold enough to attempt growing a raspberry plant in a pot indoors.  We shall see what happens*

Myricetin is a member of the flavonoid class of polyphenolic compounds with antioxidant properties.

• Has been postulated to improve cerebral metabolism,

• Protect the brain against hypoxia (low oxygen) damage and

• Scavenge free radicals

• Prevents oxidative damage

• Repairs broken DNA

• Deters cancer

• Antioxidant

This phenolic compound is prevalent in berries, vegetables, and in teas and wines produced from various plants.

**DUAL USE: Check for other benefits**

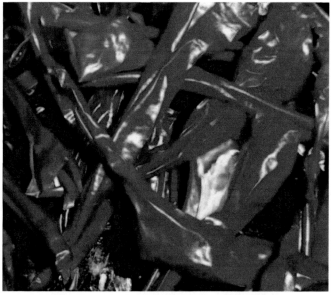

N-acetyl-cysteine (NAC)

*These peppers are paprika. Red peppers do not have to be hot. In fact, each year, I make a sweet Romanian spread called Zacusca with red peppers, eggplant, onion, olive oil, and bay leaves.*

N-acetyl-cysteine (NAC) an amino acid semi-essential because your body can produce it from other amino acids, namely methionine and serine, also a precursor of glutathione.

• Effective protector for whole-body gamma irradiation.

• Inhibits oxidative stress

• Inhibits DNA fragmentation

• Restores ovarian function

• Protects the liver against oxidative stress

Dosage: NAC administration for 7 days, 1 g NAC/kg body weight, Mansour et al.

DUAL USE:

People take N-acetyl cysteine by mouth to counteract acetaminophen (Tylenol) and carbon monoxide poisoning. It is also used for chest pain (unstable angina), genetic conditions known as lysosomal storage disorders, bile duct blockage in infants, amyotrophic lateral sclerosis (ALS, Lou Gehrig's disease), Alzheimer's disease, allergic reactions to the anti-seizure drug phenytoin (Dilantin), an eye infection called keratoconjunctivitis, and influenza symptoms. It is also used for reducing levels of a type of blood fat called lipoprotein (a), homocysteine levels (a possible risk factor for heart disease), and the risk of heart attack and stroke in people with severe kidney disease. It is also used to treat bipolar disorder, post-traumatic stress disorder (PTSD), schizophrenia, substance use disorders, and Tourette syndrome.

N-acetyl cysteine is also taken by mouth for hepatitis, kidney disease, hearing loss, ulcerative colitis, polycystic ovary syndrome (PCOS), low blood pressure, lupus, specific conditions that occur after menopause, muscle damage due to exercise, recovery after surgery, swelling of the pancreas (pancreatitis), cocaine dependence, altitude sickness, infection due to Helicobacter pylori bacteria, and for decreasing the risk for heart rhythm problems after surgery. It may also be used for genetic conditions known as adrenoleukodystrophy (ALD), erythropoietic protoporphyria (EPP), and hereditary hemorrhagic telangiectasia (HHT).

Some people use N-acetyl cysteine orally for long-term bronchitis, chronic obstructive pulmonary disease (COPD), cystic fibrosis, hay fever, human immunodeficiency virus (HIV), a lung condition called fibrosing alveolitis, autism, head and neck cancer, colorectal cancer, and lung cancer. It is also used for treating some forms of epilepsy, ear infections, complications of kidney dialysis, chronic fatigue syndrome (CFS), an autoimmune disorder called Sjogren's syndrome. It may be used for preventing sports injury complications, miscarriages, preterm labor, and liver damage due to alcohol use. Some people use N-acetyl cysteine to improve fertility and immunity to flu and H1N1 (swine) flu. It is also used for detoxifying heavy metals such as mercury, lead, and cadmium.

N-acetyl cysteine is also taken by mouth for protecting against environmental pollutants including carbon monoxide, chloroform, urethanes, and certain herbicides; reducing toxicity of drugs used for cancer treatment; reducing hearing loss caused by certain antibiotics; treating hangover symptoms; preventing kidney damage due to certain X-ray dyes, and treating compulsive hair pulling (trichotillomania).

N-acetyl cysteine is applied inside the mouth to reduce dental plaque. Also, it is used to the eye to improve dry eyes. *WebMD*

# Omega 3

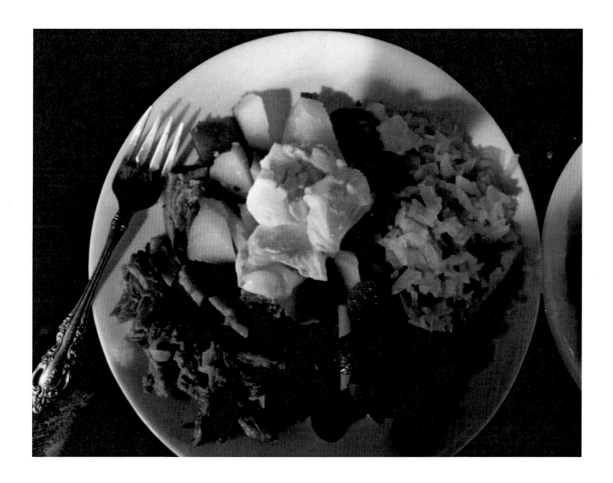

*It is very satisfying when you grow your own. This is corned elk, my own sauerkraut, fresh garden carrots, and home-grown potatoes with sour goat cream, but of course!*

**Omega 3 is a fatty acid.**

**• Radioprotective**

**• May reduce oxidative stress produced by the whole-body gamma irradiation.**

• One study that suggests the protective effects of omega-3 fatty acids on the ROS that are provided in the brain, before and during the exposure to radiation

DUAL USE: It is used for many other health conditions.

Foods with Omega 3 include:

• Fish

• Grass-Fed Beef

• Edamame

• Flaxseed Oil

• Enriched Eggs

• Walnuts

## Probiotics

The radioprotective properties of two strains of Lactobacillus Bulgaricus –LB-120 and LB-130 were used at Chernobyl:

Bifidobacterium

Probiotic bacteria Lactobacillus rhamnosus GG (LGG)

Probiotic: Armoured Acidophilus is only Lactobacillus Sporogenes product that is 100% Lactobacillus Sporigenes, the product has 30 billion live bacteria per gram (roughly 1/5th to 1/4 of a teaspoon).

At high radiation near-lethal doses, none of the gut bacteria will survive, except for maybe a few forms of E Coli. At sub-lethal doses, which is what we're being exposed to, some will do better than others. The best survivable probiotic is one that has a protective spore to keep it from harm via heat or acid. Lactobacillus sporogenes, radiation is a form of heat. Most products with this in it have it as a tiny side ingredient and not in any real quantity, and they charge an arm and leg for having it in there. Our Armoured Acidophilus is only Lactobacillus Sporogenes product that is 100% Lactobacillus Sporigenes, instead of a tiny amount.

https://drwongsessentials.com/armoured-acidophilus-survivable-acidophilus/

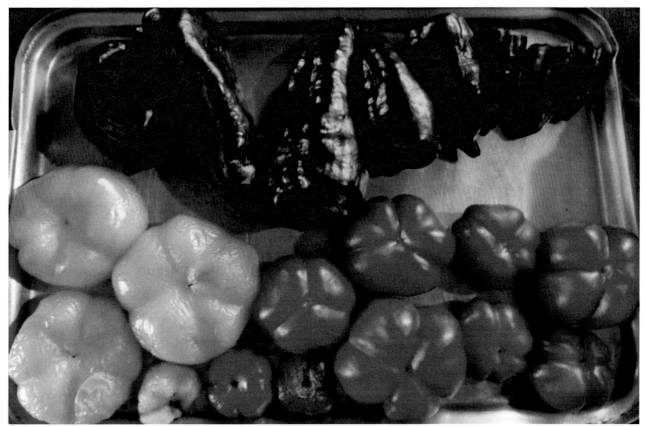

Quercetin

*These are Sheep-nose Pimentos and Poblano Peppers, which are tasty on pizza! The flavor exceeds bell peppers any day!*

Quercetin is a natural pigment present in many fruits, vegetables, and grains.

It's one of the most abundant antioxidants in the diet and plays a vital role in helping your body combat free radical damage, which is linked to chronic diseases.

• Quercetin has been postulated to improve cerebral metabolism,

• Protect the brain against hypoxia (low oxygen) damage and

• Scavenge free radicals

Foods with Quercetin: Hot yellow wax peppers, cooked onions, raw red onions, plums, fresh okra. Raw Serrano peppers, roasted asparagus, raw blueberries, raw red delicious apples, raw pears.

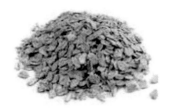

# Selenium

*My chickens get a special oatmeal on brutal Rocky Mountain winter days. It consists of oatmeal, vegetables, and cayenne pepper which warms them up and a tad of milk for calcium to keep those girls laying, which make Zippy and my egg customers happy!*

Selenium is a trace element that is naturally present in many foods and available as a dietary supplement. Selenium is a direct free radical scavenger and an indirect antioxidant via its stimulatory actions on antioxidant enzymes activity and inhibitory effects on pro-oxidative enzymes activity.

• Radioprotective of normal cells against radiation

• Antioxidant properties

• DNA repair,

• Apoptosis programmed cell death,

• Endocrine System,

• Immune systems,

• Plays a role in the prevention of cancer

• Upregulation of glutathione (GSH) and glutathione peroxidase activity

SYNERGY effect: Rostami et al. confirmed in their study that selenium and vitamin E have synergic effects, and their simultaneous administration before the exposure to X-rays provides a much more efficient protection than their separated use.

Dosage: Selenium compounds enhance the survival of irradiated mice (60Co, 0.2 Gy/min) when injected IP either before (-24 hr and -1 hr) or shortly after (+15 min) radiation exposure.

When administered at equitoxic doses (one-fourth death dose; selenomethionine = 4.0 mg/kg Se, sodium selenite = 0.8 mg/kg Se), both drugs enhanced the 30-day survival of mice irradiated at 9 Gy. Survival after 10-Gy exposure was significantly increased only after selenomethionine treatment.

An advantage of selenomethionine is lower lethal and behavioral toxicity (locomotor activity depression) compared to sodium selenite when they are administered at equivalent doses of Se.

Consideration can be given to prolonged administration of Selenium compounds for protection against long-term radiation effects.

Where is it found? Brazil nuts, brewer's yeast, wheat germ, molasses, or oil-bearing nuts. Present in fish, shellfish, and meat. The soil must be rich in selenium for plants and animals to have it. Most of the US is selenium deficient.

What is its function?

Antioxidant: Acts together with Vitamin E., Protects the cells from damage against cancer, arteriosclerosis, and degenerative diseases.

• Stimulates the immune system and contributes to the formation of antibodies against infectious agents.

• Anticarcinogen protecting against various types of cancers such as breast and skin.

• Anti-asthma

• Fertility

• Longevity

• Thyroid Function

• Lowers heart disease and inflammation

- **Boosts immunity**

- **Defends against cancer**

- **Maintains healthy eyesight**

- **Assist liver function**

- **Detoxifies**

- **Treats arthritis**

- **Treats dandruff**

**Deficiency symptoms:**

**(Selenium methionine): Essential mineral for your thyroid and your overall health. It helps reduce cancer rates when high in soil, helps boost your immune system and helps joint pain. The recommended daily dose is 200 mcg (micrograms) daily.**

**Organoselenium has radioprotective properties. Nov 01, 2009, Substances : Selenium**

**Diseases: DNA damage, Lipid Peroxidation, Radiation Induced Illness, Pharmacological Actions: Radioprotective**

# Zinc

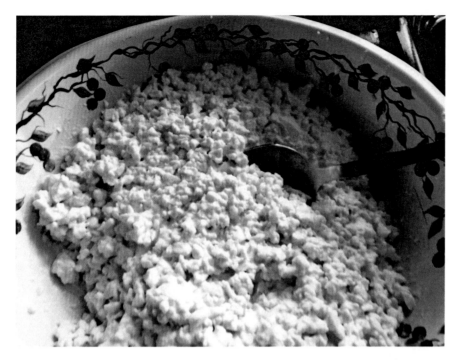

*There is nothing better than homemade cottage cheese. It is squeaky easy to make and to eat*

**What is it? Trace element**

**• Radioprotective**

**Where is it found? Meat, oysters, cured cheese, wheat germ, sesame, maple sugar, and oil-bearing nuts and legumes.**

**What is its function?**

**• Most of the zinc in the body is found in the skin, nails, hair, and prostrate. It is involved in many chemical reactions within the body since it forms various enzymes.**

**• Its primary functions include keeping the skin, hair and nails in good condition and development and functioning of the reproductive organs.**

**• Raise testosterone levels and is necessary for the production of insulin.**

**• There are several hundred enzyme systems in the body dependent upon zinc for their actions.**

- Zinc also boosts the immune system, thus its beneficial effect upon infections.

**Let's go wild!**

- Chickweed

- Curley Dock

- Dandelions

**Deficiency symptoms: Growth retardation and poor wound healing**

**When to increase it: Excess fiber consumption, pregnancy, nursing**

**Processing: Slight loss.**

**Fact checker: Oysters, meat, cheese eggs, dairy are the animal sources while plant sources are concentrated in wheat germ, sesame, maple sugar, nuts, and oats.**

**Note: Remember, if you give zinc for any length of time, you will also need to supplement with 3 mg of copper daily since zinc will lower copper levels.**

- Radioprotective

- Strengthens T-cells

**Dosage: Aim for 50 to 100 mg daily**

**Food availability: grains, nuts, seeds, and legumes.**

# Dr.Wong. Naturopath Radioprotective Suggestions

Ionizing radiation creates inflammation in your body leading to fibrosis. Radiation leads to thyroid and possible bone damage. To guard against fibrosis, use systemic enzymes is recommended. The most potent one on the planet being Zymessence or Excelzyme by AST for vegetarians.

Dosage: Zymessence dose for fibrosis and its parent inflammation is: 1 or 2 capsules taken in between meals 3x daily.

Excelzyme by AST for vegetarians,

Braggzyme by Bragg Live Foods,

W Zyme from Michael's Naturopathic Programs,

For the Thyroid: Lugol's solution

Dosage: 10 to 20 drops daily

On dosing Lugol's solution, this guide will be more exact than the numbers I gave you: https://www.iodine-resource.com/lugols-iodine.html

For the bones:

McGill University Medical School's research recommends the use plain old TUMMS as a calcium supplement and add 500 mg of ascorbic acid to 2 TUMMS tablets so that calcium ascorbate, a super well-absorbed form of calcium, is made in the gut. Each TUMMS contains 400 mg of elemental calcium (i.e., actual calcium mineral).

Magscorbate

Dosage: 1 capsule taken 2x daily for 1010 mg of elemental magnesium.

Boron: 10 mg daily.

Probiotic: Armoured Acidophilus is only Lactobacillus Sporogenes product that is 100% Lactobacillus Sporigenes, The product has 30 billion live bacteria per gram (roughly 1/5th to 1/4 of a teaspoon). https://drwongsessentials.com/armoured-acidophilus-survivable-acidophilus/

Honestly, in high near-lethal doses, none of the gut bacteria will survive, except for maybe a few forms of E Coli. At sub-lethal doses, which is what we're being exposed to some will do better than others. The best survivable probiotic is one that has a protective spore to keep it from harm via heat or acid. Lactobacillus Sporogenes, radiation being a form of heat. Most products with this in it have it as a tiny side ingredient and not in any real quantity, and they charge an arm and leg for having it in there. Our Armoured Acidophilus is only Lactobacillus Sporogenes product that is 100% Lactobacillus Sporigenes, instead of a tiny amount.

# Radio-Protective

# Foods, Herbs, and Spices

# Overview

Research on plant extracts showed that their content-polyphenols, flavones, catechins, procyanidins- has inhibitory effects on the mechanisms initiated by the X-ray and gamma-irradiation.

As you explore radioprotective foods, spices, and herbs, it is essential to note that some have synergistic potential making them work more effectively together, such as turmeric and black pepper. You get the protective power of three rather than the two individually.

Radiation induces cellular damage attributed primarily to harmful effect of free radicals, molecules with direct free radical scavenging properties are particularly promising as radiation modifiers/protectors, i.e., agents which present before or shortly after radiation exposure alter to response of tissues to radiation. Unfortunately, some of known radioprotectors are toxic at doses required for radioprotection.

The following are classifications of foods that do not neatly fit an alphabetized index:

## Fermented (Lactic acid) vegetables and juices

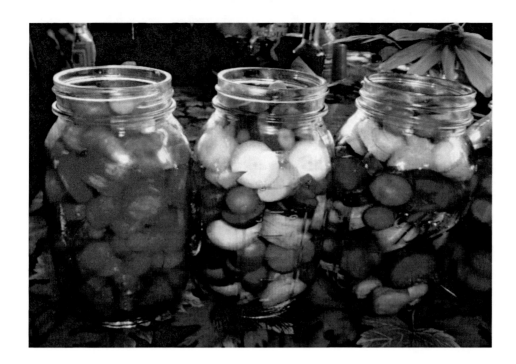

*In as little as 5 days, on your kitchen counter, you can have fermented vegetables.  Spice it up with sweet or hot pickling spices, or shredded ginger is also excellent!*

Lactic acid fermented foods possess medicinal properties and can help in the biological treatment of many conditions, including cancer, arthritis, multiple sclerosis, kidney and liver diseases, and digestive disorders. These include sauerkraut, beets, carrots, green and red pepper, beet tops, Swiss chard, and celery.

# Cultured (fermented) milk products

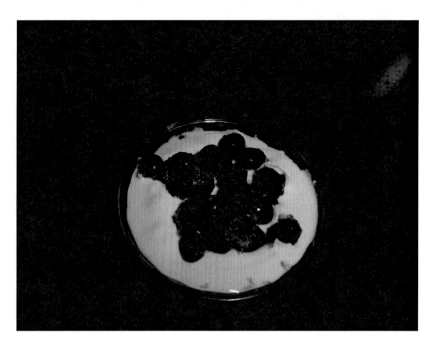

*Fresh made yogurt with your own custom probiotics is so easy to make in under 24 hours with only milk, culture, 1- 1/2 gallon thermos.  With you own berries, yum!*

Longevity studies indicate that groups of people who use cultured milk products in their diet live longer. Real yogurt is made from fresh whole (unhomogenized) milk with billions of living friendly bacteria, a minimum of honey or fructose and perhaps some real fruit. Yogurt, kefir and other fermented milks contain an unidentified substance that lowers cholesterol. Yogurt is an excellent substitute for ice cream in milkshakes and smoothies. Use it on potatoes instead of sour cream. Make your own salad dressings with yogurt, honey, vinegar and spices. These products also contain friendly bacteria, such as lactobacillus acidophilus and other strains that perform valuable duties in your colon. These bacteria colonize the colon and evict unfriendly, dangerous bacteria and other organisms from your colon. These bacteria also synthesize germ-destroying antibodies in your colon. These include yogurt, kefir, buttermilk, unprocessed cheese.

# Cruciferous vegetables

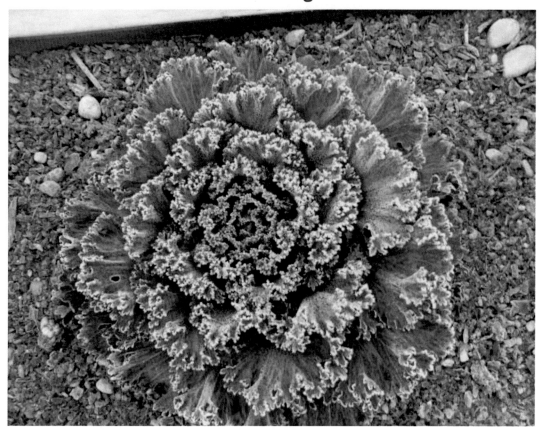

*Frost only sweetens kale up!*

This family of vegetables contain substances that inhibit breast and colon cancer cell growth. Cabbage and other cruciferous vegetables also contain dithiolthiones, a non-toxic group of compounds that have antioxidant, anticancer and anti-radiation properties. Sources include dark, leafy vegetables (broccoli, spinach, kale, Swiss chard, romaine, endive, chicory, escarole, watercress, collard, mustard and dandelion greens), dark yellow and orange vegetables (carrots, sweet potatoes, yams, pumpkins, winter squash) and fruits (cantaloupe, apricots, peaches, papayas, and watermelon).

# High-fiber foods: whole grains, fruits, and vegetables

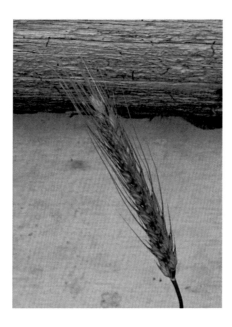

*Not quite amber waves of grain yet*

Epidemiological data suggests that a high-fiber diet protects against large bowel cancer perhaps for several reasons. It dilutes bowel carcinogens, decreases colon transit time, and changes the composition and metabolic activity of the fecal flora and certain carcinogenic substances in the colon. That's why it's healthier to eat whole grains containing the bran and the fiber, as well as whole fruits and vegetables instead of their processed, partitioned counterparts.

## Sea vegetables and their products

Sodium alginate, a non-nutritious extract from Pacific kelp used to bind and detoxify heavy metals from the body (such as lead, mercury, cadmium, etc.) and agar, used as a thickening agent instead of gelatine or corn starch, will protect the human body from radiation effects. They also reduce absorption of strontium 90 by 50-80%. Kelp and dulse, excellent natural sources of iodine, help protect against radioactive iodine, found mostly in milk. When the diet is adequately supplied with organic iodine (as in kelp), radioiodine is not as readily absorbed by the thyroid or the ovaries. Kelp contains 150,000 mcg of iodine per 100 grams (32 ounces). The RDA of iodine is 150-200 mcg. A reasonable daily dose of kelp would be 1-2 teaspoons of granules or 5-10 tablets. Other high iodine foods include seafood, beef liver, pineapple, eggs, and whole wheat. Note: Taking kelp as a source of iodine is much safer than drinking iodine or eating potassium iodide, which can be especially dangerous for pregnant women and can cause allergic reactions. Iodine (inorganic) is toxic because of its tendency to combine with protein. That's how it destroys bacteria (a protein). When you put iodine into your mouth, it combines with the protein there and in your stomach or wherever it goes. This causes irritation or worse. Also, sudden large doses of iodine in humans with a normal thyroid may reduce the synthesis of thyroid hormone.

## Essential fatty acids

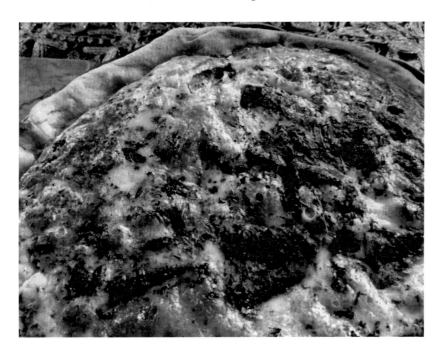

*One of my favorite past times with David was salmon fishing. Those red salmon are truly fighters.*

GLA and EPA EFAs are essential for proper functioning of the immune system and protect against cancer. Food sources include flaxseed oil, evening primrose oil and certain fish, particularly salmon. Information for this report was excerpted from Fighting Radiation and Chemical Pollutants with Foods, Herbs and Vitamins, by Steven Schecter, N.D., and Radiation Protection Manual, Lita Lee, Ph.D.

This guide is alphabetized for your convenience. Some plants include their Latin and common names.

I highly recommend purchasing two complimentary reference manuals for your libraries:

Physicians' Desk Reference, <u>PDR Herbal Medicine</u>.

This book provides usage, dosage, precautions, contraindications, and peer studies for all your favorite herb, spices, and foods. Cost is between $3-60 depending on publication date and whether it is used or new.

<u>Physicians Desk Reference</u>, PDR for Notional Supplements. This book provides usage, dosage, precautions, contraindications, and peer studies for all your favorite supplements. Cost is between $19-50 depending on publication date and whether it is used or new.

# Remember!

## Always check with your health care physician

and these reference for contraindications for when NOT to consume foods, herbs, spices, or supplements.

## Be aware most physicians are not trained in nutrition

and may not know if a supplement, herb, spice, or food may interact with a current health care condition, synergistic interactions, allegories, or current cosmic storms.

## Growing your own is always recommended.

The supply chain for imported items may become disrupted because of various means in the days to come.

# Radio-Protective Supplements to Purchase

# Radio-Protective Foods, Spices, and Herbs

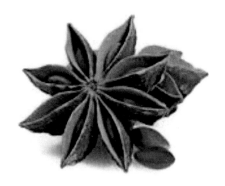

## Illicium verum, known as, Star Anise

*Anise tastes like licorice and can be used to make delicious bran crackers, as a spice for pickling, or to be used to create exotic beverages*

Illicium verum, commonly known as Star Anise. The essential oil has confectionary application as a flavoring agent and industrial application in the preparation of Tamiflu to act against influenza virus. Anisyl acetone and benzene carboxylic acid were identified as the main phenolic components present in aqueous fraction of I. verum. I. verum extract showed radioprotective effects in irradiated minced chicken meat by reducing lipid peroxidation. It is an antioxidant.

## Ageratum conyzoides, known as, Billy Goat Weed

The plant Ageratum belongs to the family Asteraceae, which consists of about 30 species. The name is derived from the Greek word 'a geras' and konyz, referring to extended life and similarity with Inula helenium. The weed is best known for its healing activity and has been used for treating burn, wound, skin diseases, and various infections, among others, since ancient times. Ageratum conyzoides contains multiple chemical constituents. It is rich in polyoxygenated flavonoids. It is radioprotective.

Dose: An optimum dose of 75 mg/kg was found to be effective against radiation doses ranging from 6 to 11 Gy and resulted in reduction in gastrointestinal- and bone marrow-associated death in mice. In vitro studies showed A. conyzoides extract was also effective in scavenging DPPH radicals suggesting free radical scavenging mechanism of radioprotection.

## Aegle marmelos Correa, known as, Bael

The hydroalcoholic extract of Aegle marmelos (AME) protected cultured HPBLs against the radiation-induced micronuclei at a concentration of 5 μg/ml. It was also reported to scavenge ·OH, O2·–, DPPH, ABTS·+ and NO (nitric oxide) radicals in vitro in a concentration-dependent manner.

Dose: The radioprotective efficacy of 15 or 250 mg/kg AME was further confirmed in animal studies where its intraperitoneal, as well as oral administration, has been found to protect mice against the radiation-induced sickness, gastrointestinal and bone marrow deaths and mortality giving a DRF of 1.2. It also protected mice against the radiation-induced lipid peroxidation and elevated GSH concentration in the liver, kidney, stomach and intestine at 31 days post-irradiation. Oral administration also protected mice against the gamma radiation-induced decline in erythrocytes, leukocytes, lymphocytes and clonogenicity of hemopoietic progenitor cells assessed by exogenous spleen colony-forming assay.

Not only leaf but also the hydroalcoholic extract of Aegle marmelos fruit administered intraperitoneally at a dose of 20 mg/kg once daily, consecutively for five days found to protect mice against the radiation-induced sickness, gastrointestinal as well as bone marrow deaths with a DRF of 1.1.

When: Pre-treatment of mice with AME elevated the villus height and the crypt number accompanied by a decline in goblet and dead cell number.

Aegle marmelos (Bael) has radioprotective properties. Oct 01, 2010

Pharmacological Actions: Antineoplastic Agents, Chemopreventive, Chemoprotective Agents, Radioprotective

# Aloe

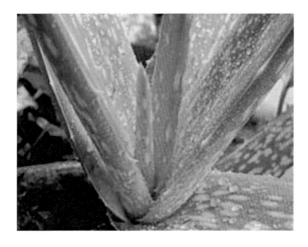

*Did you know that there are many varieties of aloe with different constituents? I love to include aloe in my DIY shampoo bars!*

Aloe barbadensis can play a significant role in dentistry in treatment of lichen planus, oral submucous fibrosis, recurrent aphthous stomatitis, alveolar osteitis, periodontitis. Mar 31, 2015

Diseases: Gingivitis, Lichen Planus, Oral Submucous Fibrosis, Periodontal Diseases, Radiation-Induced Illness: Mucositis, Stomatitis: Aphthous

Pharmacological Actions: Anti-Bacterial Agents, Anti-Inflammatory Agents, Immunomodulatory, Radioprotective

## Amaranth

Dose: Daily oral administration of 800 mg/kg body weight (b. wt.) of Rajgira (Amaranthus paniculatus) leaf extract for 15 consecutive days before whole-body exposure to $\gamma$-radiation protected mice against the radiation-induced lethality with a dose reduction factor of 1.36. Rajgara extract also arrested radiation-induced lipid peroxidation and the decline in reduced glutathione in the liver and blood of mice.

# Apple Pectin

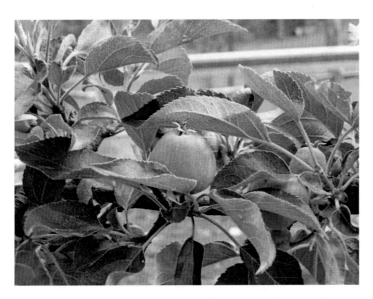

*I grow many types of apple trees, many in containers, but my favorite is my espalier apple tree*

From 1996 to 2007, a total of more than 160,000 "Chernobyl" children received pectin food additives. As a result, levels of Cs-137 in children's organs decreased after each course of pectin additives by an average of 30-40%. Apr 01, 2009

Substances: Apple Pectin, Diseases: Radiation Disaster Associated Toxicity, Radiation-Induced Illness: Cesium-137 Exposure, Pharmacological Actions: Detoxifier, Radioprotective

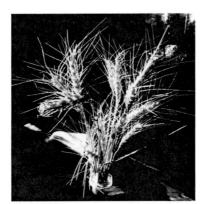

Barley (wheat) grass

*Next year's wheatgrass, but now, a lovely fall decoration to enjoy!*

Barley is a totally balanced food. It contains all the nutrients required for life: vitamins, minerals, enzymes and other proteins (amino acids), essential fatty acids and chlorophyll. Barley grass has thousands of living enzymes (a unique protein). Enzymes are nature's biological catalysts that initiate all the chemical transformations in the body. Over 3,000 enzymes have been identified. They are required for every change in the body - digestion, cell respiration, bodily movements, thinking processes, detoxification, cancer control, fat, protein, and carbohydrate metabolism, etc.

Dose: The average daily amount of barley grass is 1-3 teaspoons (1 tsp = 2 grams). If you choose wheatgrass (juice), start with one ounce daily and gradually increase to four or six ounces.

## Aegle marmelos Correa, known as, Bael

Dose: The hydroalcoholic extract of Aegle marmelos (AME) protected cultured HPBLs.

Not only leaf but also the hydroalcoholic extract of Aegle marmelos fruit administered intraperitoneally at a dose of 20 mg/kg once daily, consecutively for five days found to protect mice against the radiation-induced sickness, gastrointestinal as well as bone marrow deaths with a DRF of 1.1 against the radiation-induced micronuclei at a concentration of 5 µg/ml.

It was also reported to scavenge ·OH, O2·–, DPPH, ABTS·+ and NO (nitric oxide) radicals in vitro in a concentration-dependent manner. The radioprotective efficacy of 15 or 250 mg/kg AME was further confirmed in animal studies where its intraperitoneal, as well as oral administration, has been found to protect mice against the radiation-induced sickness, gastrointestinal and bone marrow deaths and mortality giving a DRF of 1.2. It also protected mice against the radiation-induced lipid peroxidation and elevated GSH concentration in the liver, kidney, stomach and intestine at 31 days post-irradiation.

Oral administration also protected mice against the gamma radiation-induced decline in erythrocytes, leukocytes, lymphocytes and clonogenicity of hemopoietic progenitor cells assessed by exogenous spleen colony-forming assay.

When: Pre-treatment of mice with AME elevated the villus height and the crypt number accompanied by a decline in goblet and dead cell number.

## Basil

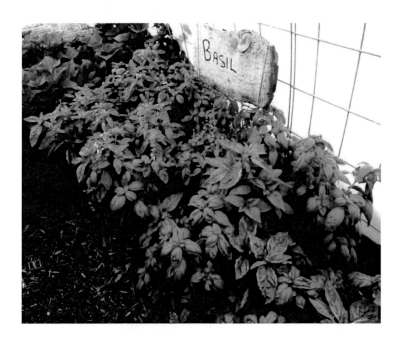

*Basil is so flexible and with so many different tastes!  Grow some in your kitchen garden.  My favorite dish is Pesto.*

Ocimum species have anti-melanoma and radioprotective activity against metastatic melanoma cell line-induced metastasis. Mar 31, 2011

Substances: African Basil, Basil

Diseases: Malignant Melanoma, Melanoma: Metastatic

Pharmacological Actions: Anti-metastatic, Radioprotective

## Ageratum conyzoides, known as, Billy Goat Weed

The plant Ageratum belongs to the family Asteraceae, which consists of about 30 species. The name is derived from the Greek word 'a geras' and konyz, referring to long life and similarity with Inula helenium. The weed is best known for its healing activity and has been used for treating burn, wound, skin diseases, and various infections, among others, since ancient times. Ageratum conyzoides contains various chemical constituents. It is rich in polyoxygenated flavonoids. It is radioprotective.

Dose: An optimum dose of 75 mg/kg was found to be effective against radiation doses ranging from 6 to 11 Gy and resulted in reduction in gastrointestinal- and bone marrow-associated death in mice. In vitro studies showed A. conyzoides extract was also effective in scavenging DPPH radicals suggesting free radical scavenging mechanism of radioprotection.

## Citrus aurantium, known as, Bitter Orange

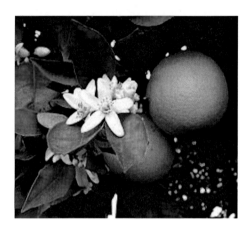

*For me, these bring back fond memories of my maternal grandmother, who grew them alongside her driveway. They are very popular in the Persian culture in cooking*

Citrus aurantium. The essential oil of Bitter Orange possesses antianxiety and motor relaxant effects in rats and mice. The main flavonoids occurring in cultivated citrus species are flavanone glycosides, hesperidin and naringin, accounting for 5% of dry weight of leaves and fruits. These exhibit potent antioxidant activity.

Dose: Citrus extract at different doses (250, 500, and 1000 mg/kg) have shown radioprotective effects against 1.5 Gy γ-irradiation in mouse bone marrow; however, 250 mg/kg dose was found to be the optimum dose, providing 2.2-fold protection. Radioprotective activity was assigned to the flavonoids contained in citrus extract.

## Syzygium cumini, known as, Black Plums

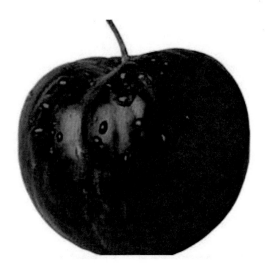

*My Black Plum tree will bear fruit next year. I am so excited! Fruit trees take at least 4 years to bear fruit after planting*

Black Plum or Skeels, Syzygium cumini. Skeels are also known as Eugenia cumini (family Myrtaceae) and has been reported to possess several medicinal properties in the folklore system of medicine. The micronucleus study of radioprotective effect of dichloromethane and methanol (1:1) extract of jamun (SCE) in human peripheral blood lymphocytes (HPBLs).

Dosage: Radioprotective potential, where 12.5 µg/ml SCE was found to reduce the micronuclei up to a maximum extent. In vivo evaluation further established its radioprotective activity where it was found to reduce radiation-induced sickness, gastrointestinal, and bone marrow deaths.

Not only leaf but the hydroalcoholic extract of jamun seeds (JSE) also exhibited a most significant protective effect at 80 mg/kg JSE. The JSE was more effective when administered through the intraperitoneal route at equimolar doses than the oral. The JSE treatment protected mice against the gastrointestinal as well as bone marrow deaths with a DRF of 1.24

# Nigella sativa, known as Love in the Mist or Black Seed

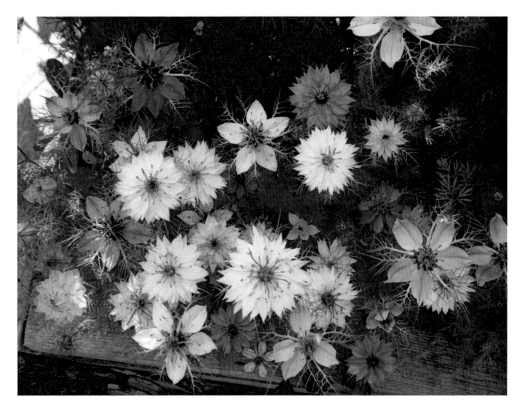

*What isn't there to love about Love in the Mist? Garden beauty, health, and unique pods for exquisite bouquets, and radio-protective!*

Nigella sativa belongs to the family Ranunculaceae and is commonly called black seed. The most important active compounds of black seeds are thymoquinone, thymohydroquinone, dithymoquinone, p-cymene, carvacrol, 4-terpineol, t-anethol, sesquiterpene longifolene αpinene and thymol among others. Seeds also contain alkaloids as isoquinoline and pyrazole ring bearing alkaloids. Additionally, N. Sativa seeds contain αhederin, a water-soluble pentacyclic triterpene and saponin.

Radioprotection by N. sativa extract and oil was studied in mice and rats. The extract of N. Sativa was evaluated in mice to assess protection against radiation-induced damage. Nigella sativa extract treatment showed significant reduction in lipid peroxidation and intracellular reactive oxygen species in splenocytes and increased the survival rate of irradiated animals, suggesting a radioprotective potential of N. Sativa.

When: Oral administration of N. Sativa oil before irradiation resulted in significant increase in blood malondialdehyde, nitrate and nitrite levels and antioxidant enzymes.

# Black Tea

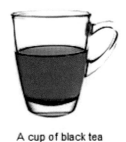

A cup of black tea

**Containing tannin and honey is used for radiation protection in China.**

## Buckwheat

**buckwheat extract has antioxidant and photoprotective properties. Mar 01, 2006**

**Diseases: Oxidative Stress, Skin Diseases: Photo-Aging, Sunburn**

**Pharmacological Actions: Antioxidants, Radioprotective**

**Additional Keywords: Plant Extracts**

## Theobroma Cacao, known as, Cocoa powder

*The darker and less refined you can get it, the better.  I wish you could grow cocoa indoors, but you probably would not get any cocoa pods.  Sorry...*

**Dosage: Late radiation effects after whole-body gamma-radiation in rats were inhibited by increasing the activity of antioxidant enzymes. 1 g cocoa powder/kg for 21 days**

The radioprotective effects of sulforaphane, an Nrf2 inducer identified in cruciferous vegetables (broccoli, Brussels sprouts, cabbages), were studied by Mathew et al. on human skin fibroblasts. The study showed that sulforaphane has dose-dependent effects and may protect against ionizing radiation damages if it is administered repeatedly before the fibroblast exposure. It is an antioxidant.

Elettaria cordamomum is commonly called cardamom and belongs to the family Zingiberaceae. The volatile oil contains about 1.5% α-pinene, 0.2% β-pinene, 2.8% sabinene, 1.6% myrcene, 0.2% α-phellandrene, 11.6% limonene, 36.3% 1,8-cineole, 0.7% γ-terpinene, 0.5% terpinolene, 3% linalool, 2.5% linalyl acetate, 0.9% terpinen 4-ol, 2.6% α-terpineol, 31.3% α-terpinyl acetate, 0.3% citronellol, 0.5% nerd, 0.5% geraniol, 0.2% methyl eugenol and 2.7% trans-nerolidol.

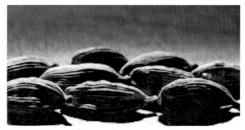
Cardamom

*I use Cardamom in almost everything from a season various dishes and in making my delicious Ginger, Rose Water Lemon, Cardamom Soda with honey, and a pinch of cayenne!*

Has been evaluated for its radioprotective effects against γ-irradiation in rats and found to afford protection against radiation-induced oxidative damage in liver and heart tissues. No dosage was mentioned.

# Citrus Extract

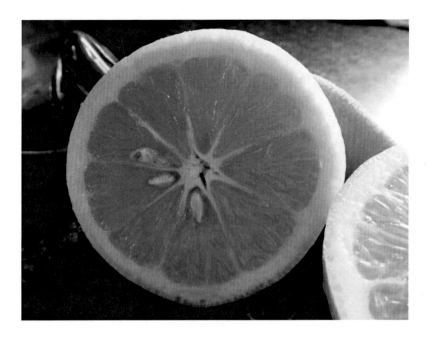

*It is easy to make your own citrus extract! Use the peels and put them in Vodka, Everclear or Glycerine. In about 6 months, you have whatever flavor extract you desire! This is from a windowsill Meyer Lemon*

**Citrus extract protects against gamma irradiation-induced toxicity in bone marrow cells. Sep 01, 2003**

**Substances: Citrus Peel, Diseases: Radiation-Induced Illness, Radiation-Induced Illness: Bone Marrow, Pharmacological Actions: Antiproliferative, Radioprotective**

## Chlorophyll

**Foods containing chlorophyll: barley grass and chlorella. Chlorophyll closely resembles human blood and is used to cleanse, detoxify, purify and heal many conditions. It retards bacterial growth, detoxifies heavy metals from the body, increases wound healing, detoxifies the liver and other organs, deodorizes the body, removes putrefactive bacteria from the colon, aids healing of 11 types of skin diseases, relieves ulcers, gastritis, pancreatitis, and other inflammatory conditions, helps heal gum diseases and the metabolic activation of many carcinogens. It is radioprotective. No dosage mentioned.**

## Chlorella

**Is a green freshwater micro-It is algae which has even more chlorophyll than barley (wheat) grass plus 55-65% protein with 19 amino acids, including all the essential ones? It's an excellent source of beta-carotene, vitamins B-I, B-2, B-3,**

B-6, B-12, pantothenic acid, folic acid, biotin, PABA, inositol and vitamin C. Contains essential minerals - iron, phosphorus, magnesium, calcium, zinc, potassium, sulfur, and iodine with trace amounts of manganese, sodium and chlorine.

## Cherries (sweet)

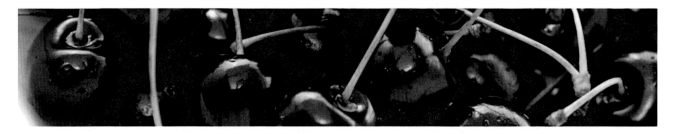

*Dark Sweet Cherries are world-famous in my area. I just pitted and processed 100 pounds in under 24 hours. My personal record! My reward? Taste and radioprotection!*

An ultrasound-assisted extract of sweet cherry seemed to act as a radioprotector at lower doses and a radiosensitizer at higher doses. Feb 28, 2018

**Pharmacological Actions: Antioxidants, Radioprotective, Radiosensitizer**

**Additional Keywords: Plant Extracts**

## Chicory

An extract of chicory seeds had radio-protective effects in vitro. Dec 31, 2014

**Pharmacological Actions: Antioxidants, Radioprotective**

**Anti-Therapeutic Actions: Low Dose Ionizing Radiation**

## Syzygium aromaticum, known as, Clove

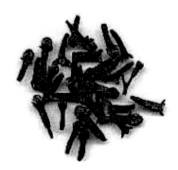

*Did you know that cloves can stop some of the pain from a toothache?  It is a pioneer remedy and if you get a root canal, your dentist uses a form of clove oil.*

Syzygium aromaticum or Eugenia caryophyllata and Eugenia aromaticum. Clove oil is applied externally for relieving pain and promotes healing. The main constituents of the essential oil are phenylpropanoids such as carvacrol, thymol, eugenol and cinnamaldehyde.

The radioprotective effect of clove oil has been studied in rats on specific biochemical parameters against ionizing radiation. It has been demonstrated that the radioprotective effects of clove oil may be assigned to its capacity to reduce lipid peroxidation, strong reducing power, and superoxide radical scavenging activity owing to presence of the polyphenol as well as trace element contents.

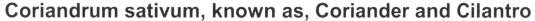

Coriandrum sativum, known as, Coriander and Cilantro

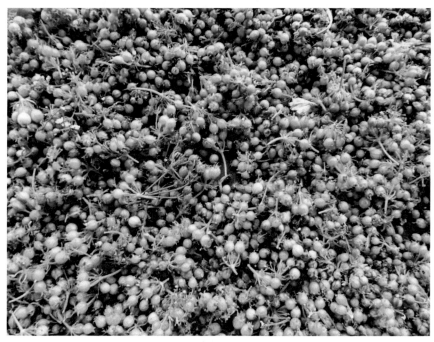

*Cilantro makes your salsa but you can also use it in salads, wraps, and in casseroles. Make sure you check for slow bolting varieties to have a more extended cilantro season. Once it seeds, it is known as Coriander. I love coriander. Good thing now that we need radioprotection!*

Coriandrum sativum L. belongs to the family Umbelliferae (Apiaceae), commonly called as coriander. Phytochemical constituents of C. sativum seeds showed the presence of polyphenols (rutin, caffeic acid derivatives, ferulic acid, gallic acid and chlorogenic acid), flavonoids (quercetin and isoquercetin) and β-carotenoids. Seeds of coriander mainly contain essential oils; however, leaves contain caffeic acid and flavonoids apart from volatile oils.

The radioprotective effect of coriander seeds against whole-body γ-irradiation was studied in rats. Treatment with coriander seed extract was effective in preventing radiation-induced biochemical changes in serum and significantly improved the antioxidant status in liver and kidney of rats. It is suggested that scavenging of free radicals was a possible mechanism of protection. Ethanol extract of C. sativum was effective against Ultraviolet B (UVB)-induced skin photoaging in vitro and in vivo. Thinner epidermal layers and denser dermal collagen fibers was observed in treated mice, which also had lower MMP-1 levels and higher procollagen type I levels, thus suggesting the ability of C. sativum extract to prevent UVB-induced skin photoaging.

## Crocus sativus, known as, Saffron or Autumn Crocus

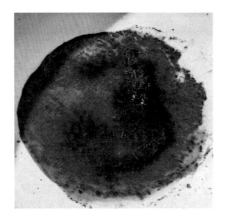

*I use saffron to color my cuisine. My favorite is a Persian Wedding Hen with rice pilaf and a variety of dried fruits draped with the Saffron and Honey Sauce! Great for company!*

Crocus sativus L. belongs to family Iridaceae. The significant components of saffron are cis- and trans-crocins, which are glucosyl esters of 8,8'-diapocarotene-8,8'-dioic acid (crocetin), one of the few families of carotenoids that are freely soluble in water. It also contains safranal, which is a monoterpene aldehyde, and picrocrocin, which is a glycosidic precursor of safranal. Saffron is known to carry around 150 volatile and aromatic compounds including terpenes, terpene alcohol, and their esters.

When: Pre-treatment with freeze-dried saffron extract resulted in significant protective effects against radiation-induced genotoxic damage in mouse bone marrow; it reduced the level of lipid peroxidation and resulted in an increase in glutathione content and activity of glutathione S-transferase, glutathione peroxidase and catalase liver and brain tissues of mice. There is insignificant intestinal protection.

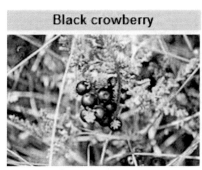

Black crowberry

Crowberry

Empetrum nigrum var. japonicum extract suppresses γ-ray radiation-induced cell damage via inhibition of oxidative stress. Dec 31, 2010

Substances: Crowberry

Diseases: DNA damage, Lipid Peroxidation, Oxidative Stress, Radiation-Induced Illness

Pharmacological Actions: Antioxidants, Radioprotective

Additional Keywords: Plant Extracts

# Catchin and or Chamomile

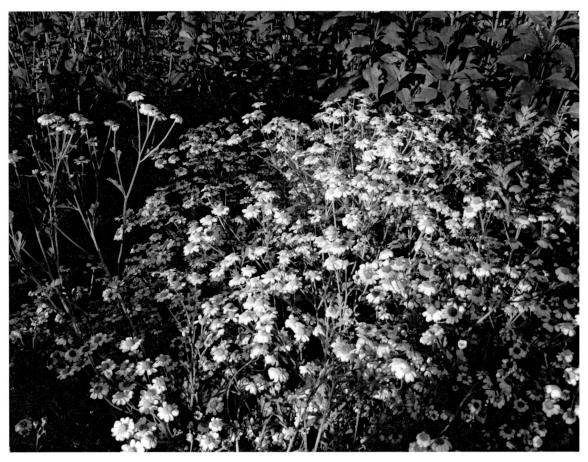

*There are various varieties of Chamomile.  Some, when extracted, exudes a vibrant indigo-blue essential oil that is exceptionally anti-inflammatory and smells heavenly!*

This literature review discusses the topical agents studied for the treatment of acute radiation dermatitis. Feb 21, 2019

Click here to read the entire abstract

Substances: Aloe Vera, Catechin, Chamomile, Marigold, Vitamin C

Diseases: Chemotherapy and Radiation Toxicity, Dermatitis

Pharmacological Actions: Radioprotective

# Cruciferous vegetables

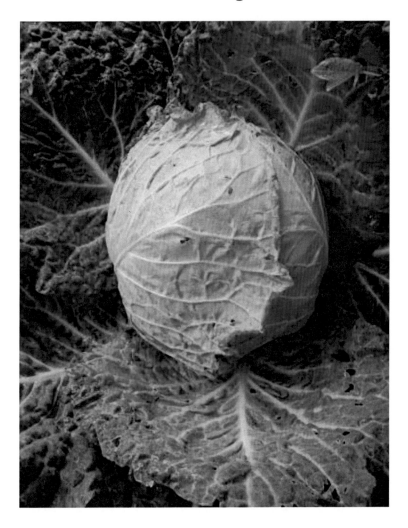

*The Cabbage Patch will provide you with good food in cold climates. They thrive on cold and wet. Explore other cultures to see how they use their cruciferous vegetables.*

The radioprotective effects of sulforaphane, an Nrf2 inducer identified in cruciferous vegetables (broccoli, Brussels sprouts, cabbages), were studied by Mathew et al. on human skin fibroblasts. The study showed that sulforaphane has dose-dependent effects and may protect against ionizing radiation damages.

When: Administered repeatedly before the fibroblast exposure

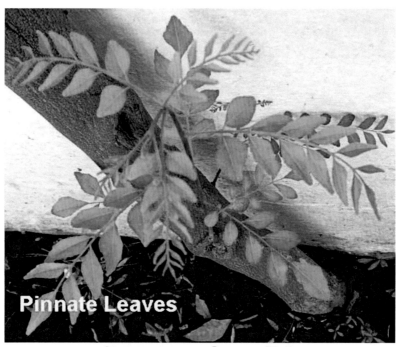

, known as, Curry Tree

**Murraya koenigii L. belongs to the family Rutaceae and is commonly known as Meethi neem or curry-leaf. Leaves are aromatic and contain proteins, carbohydrates, fiber, minerals, carotene, nicotinic acid and vitamin C. The leaves contain high amount of oxalic acid and also contain crystalline glycosides, carbazole alkaloids, koenigin and resin. Fresh leaves contain yellow-colored volatile oil that is also rich in vitamin A and calcium. It also contains girinimbin, iso-mahanimbin, koenine, koenigine, koenidine and koenimbine. Mahanimbicine, bicyclomahanimbicine, phebalosin, coumarin as murrayone imperatoxin etc. are isolated from leaves. Triterpenoid alkaloids-cyclomahanimbine and tetrahydromahanmbine are present in the leaves. Alkaloids-murrayastine, murrayaline, pypayafolinecarbazole have been reported in the leaves of M. koenigii.**

**The radioprotective effect of M. koenigii leaf extract was evaluated against 4 Gy γ-irradiation in liver. The leaf extract itself was useful for significantly increasing reduced glutathione (GSH) content and antioxidant enzyme levels in liver as well as it reduced the radiation-induced decrease in lipid peroxidation, thus indicating the antioxidant properties of extract possibly contributing for radioprotection.**

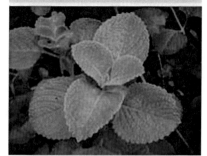

*Plectranthus amboinicus*

Coleus aromaticus

Coleus aromaticus, belonging to family Lamiaceae, is native to India and the Mediterranean and possesses various medicinal values. The report on the chemical constituents of the leaves of C. aromaticus indicated the presence of carvacrol, thymol, eugenol, chavicol, ethyl salicylate, chlorophyllin, flavonoids (cirsimaritin) and β-sitosterol-β-D-glucoside.

Radioprotective potential was evaluated for C. aromaticus extract. In cell-free assay, the extract has been shown to have radical scavenging activity and in V79 cells frequencies of micronuclei were evaluated against 0.5, 1, 2 and 4 Gy doses of γ-radiation. Both the assays demonstrated that the extract had antioxidant, anticlastogenic, and radioprotective properties.

# Dates

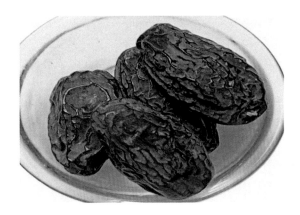

*Dates are fabulous for health from radioprotection to high fiber. My ideal date recipe is a good date shake with a sprinkle of nutmeg on top!*

**When: Pre-treatment of rats with Date syrup ameliorated the tissue damage induced by radiation as evidenced by the improvement of liver function, antioxidant status, and reduction of DNA damage.**

**Date pits effective against gamma radiation.**

**Water extract of date pit extract may have an ameliorative effect on gamma radiation toxicity. Jul 02, 2018**

Allium sativum, known as, Garlic

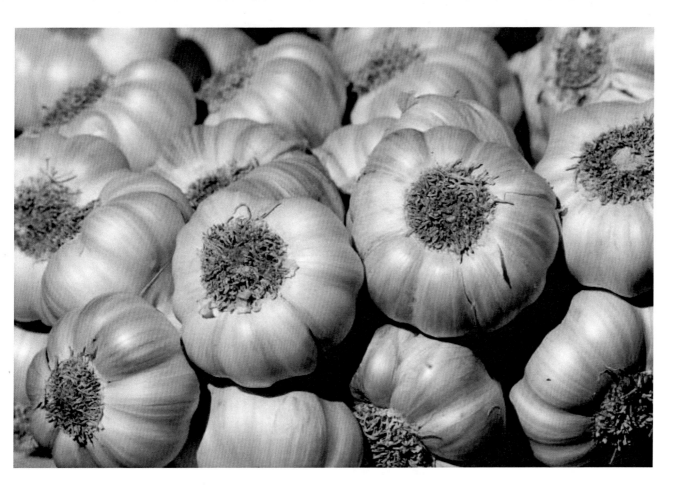

*Garlic is easy to grow. Make sure that you save some of your harvest haul for seed stock the next year. Store it in a cool, dark place. I store my garlic in a burlap bap. Back in the days before keto Garlic Bread was my favorite!*

**Allium sativum L. belongs to the genus Allium. It is rich in c-glutamylcysteine and other sulfur-containing compounds giving a characteristic flavor. However, additional constituents of garlic include a wide range of primary and secondary non-sulfur biomolecules, such as steroidal glycosides, essential oil, flavonoids, anthocyanins, lectins, prostaglandins, fructan, pectin, adenosine, vitamins B1, B2, B6, C and E, biotin, nicotinic acid, fatty acids, glycolipids, phospholipids, and essential amino acids.**

**A. sativum extract has demonstrated radioprotective effects in mice and was found to be effective in significantly reducing the micronuclei frequencies induced by radiation.**

**Dose notations: A dose-dependent effect was evaluated on the frequencies of damaged cells and chromosomal aberrations, and it was recommended that**

administration of the extract for 30 days is vital for mitigating the clastogenic effects of genotoxicants.

Necessary notation: Recent investigations showed that aged garlic is superior to fresh garlic as far as antiglycation and antioxidant activities are concerned.

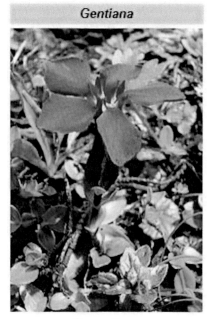

Gentian

*The flower is more vibrant than this but it gives you an idea. It has many uses, including being an old-time remedy for thrush (fungus).*

Gentiana lutea extract and mangiferin have radioprotective activities. Nov 01, 2010

Substances: Gentian, Mangiferin, Diseases: Radiation-Induced Illness

Pharmacological Actions: Radioprotective, Additional Keywords: Plant Extracts, Xanthones

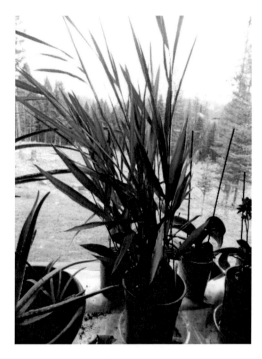

Ginger

*Some of my ginger a few years ago. Now I have a jungle of ginger. I love my DIY Ginger Soda!*

**Ameliorative and protective effects of ginger and its main constituents against natural, chemical, and radiation-induced toxicities. Oct 21, 2018**

**Diseases: Chemotherapy and Radiation Toxicity**

**Pharmacological Actions: Anti-Inflammatory Agents, Antioxidants, Chemoprotective Agents, Radioprotective**

Ginseng

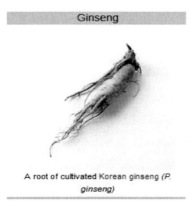

A root of cultivated Korean ginseng (P. ginseng)

*I have not attempted to grow ginseng, but maybe I should give it a try!*

**American ginseng protects human peripheral lymphocytes from radiation-induced oxidative stress. Jan 01, 2009**

**Diseases: DNA damage, Radiation-Induced Illness, Radiation-Induced Illness: Cesium-137 Exposure,**

**Pharmacological Actions: Radioprotective**

**American ginseng reduces genotoxicity lymphocytes after Cesium irradiation. Jan 10, 2004**

**Diseases: Radiation-Induced Illness, Radiation-Induced Illness: Cesium-137 Exposure**

**Pharmacological Actions: Radioprotective**

**Additional Keywords: Plant Extracts**

## Grapeseed Extract (GSE)

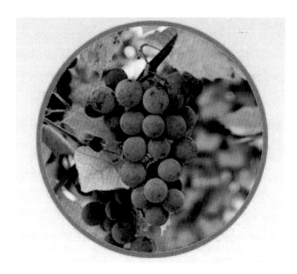

Grapevines are hardy to -30 (some varieties). Keep the grapes on the vine until after a frost or two to sweeten up grapes. The leaves are eatable and one of my favorites are Stuffed Grape Leaves!

Singha et al. suggested that grape seed extract administered in high concentration, maybe a potent protector through its antioxidant effects against low dose of ionizing radiation. Grape seed extract contains phenols that initiate the synthesis of liver antioxidants.

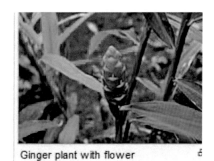

Ginger plant with flower

Zingiber officinale, known as, Ginger

*I have yet to get my ginger plants to flower....someday....sigh!*

Zingiber officinale is commonly called ginger and belongs to the family Zingiberaceae. The essential oil possesses antibacterial, antifungal and antiviral activities. Antioxidant, anti-inflammatory and antinociceptive properties have also been reported. Gingerol-related compounds such as gingerol, shagaols, gengediols, zingerone, dehydrozingerone, gingerinone and diarylheptanoids accord antioxidant capacity to the ginger rhizome. Geranial, camphene, p-cineole, α-terpineole, zingiberene and petandeconoic acid were the major components of the essential oil.

Radioprotective effects of ginger extract were demonstrated in rats exposed to X-irradiation on the liver, kidney and heart. Results indicated that ginger extract had significant anti-radiation activity. Antioxidant status and antioxidant enzymes were studied in rats with pretreatment of ginger extract and whole-body irradiated with γ-radiation. Hematological parameters were found to have significant recovery concerning radiation-induced damage. Essential oil of ginger was also evaluated for its radioprotective effects in mice, yielding a dose reduction factor of 1.4. Ginger oil was found to be effective in restoring antioxidant status and reducing the cytogenetic damage in terms of chromosomal aberrations, micronuclei frequency, and DNA damage in mice.

Dosage: Administration of 10 mg/kg (i.p) or 250 mg/kg (orally) hydroalcoholic extract once daily, consecutively for 5 days was found to protect mice against the radiation-sickness, gastrointestinal as well as bone marrow deaths with a DRF of 1.15. Ginger has been reported to increase glutathione, reduce lipid peroxidation in vivo and scavenging of various free radicals in vitro].

## Withania somnifera, known as, Indian Ginseng

Withania somnifera, belonging to the family Solanaceae and popularly known as Indian ginseng or ashwagandha. The extract of W. somnifera is a complex mixture of several phytochemicals, including phenolic compounds and flavonoids. However, the pharmacological effect of the roots of W. somnifera is attributed to withanolides.

The protective effects of root extract of W. somnifera against radiation-induced oxidative stress and DNA damage in liver were investigated in rats.

When: Withania, somnifera treatment prior to radiation exposure, showed significant decrease in hepatic enzymes, hepatic nitrate/nitrite ratio, MDA levels and DNA damage. Also, considerable increase in heme oxygenase activity, superoxide dismutase, glutathione peroxidase activities, and glutathione content suggest a possible role of W. somnifera as a radioprotective.

The radioprotective efficacy of ginseng (Panax ginseng) has been reported by several workers. Ginseng treatment caused recovery of thrombocyte, and erythrocyte counts in blood after irradiation.

Water-soluble whole extract of ginseng provided best protection against radiation-induced damage in C3H mice, whereas isolated protein and carbohydrate fractions were less effective. The saponin fraction was ineffective. Similar results were obtained by Kim and coworkers, who found that whole ginseng extract and its fractions increased endogenous spleen colony formation in irradiated mice and also reduced apoptosis in jejunal crypt cells. The radioprotective effect of ginseng root extract on testicular enzymes-acid and alkaline phosphatases and lipid peroxidation has also been reported. It is a protective agent through antioxidant function and heme oxygenase induction.

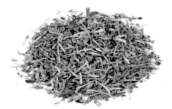

Centella asiatica, also known as, Asiatic pennywort or Gotu Kola

Centella asiatica belongs to family Umbelliferae (Apiaceae). It contains triterpenoids such as asiatcoside, centelloside, madecossoside, thankuniside, isothankunic acid, centellose, asiatic, centellic and madecassic acids. The other constituents includes brahmoside, brahminoside and brahmic acid. The fatty oil consists of glycerides of palmitic, stearic, lignoceric, oleic, linoleic and linolenic acids. An alkaloid, hydrocotylin, has been isolated from the dried plants. Asiaticoside, madecossoside and centelloside have been isolated from the plant parts. Flavanoids, 3-glucosylquercetin, 3-glucosylkaemferol and 7-glucosylkaemferol have been isolated from the leaves.

Dosage: C. asiatica extract at 100 mg/kg body weight was effective in mice against radiation (8 Gy)-induced loss in body weight, and in survival. It was reported that C. asiatica offered protection against radiation to DNA as well as membranes. The proposed mechanism for this was by antioxidant function.

Aqueous extract of Centella asiatica reduced the adverse effect of low dose irradiation in Sprague Dawley rats by inhibiting radiation-induced body weight loss and conditioned taste aversion. Similarly, it has been found to protect against the radiation-induced weight loss in mice exposed to 8 Gy $\gamma$-radiations.

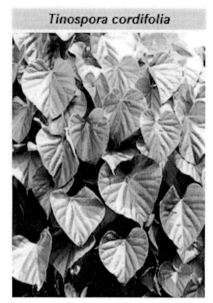

Tinospora cordifolia

Heart-Leaved Moonseed, known as, Guduchi, Guduchi, and giloy

Oral administration of an aqueous extract of Guduchi, Tinospora cordifolia has been reported to increase the survival of mice exposed to radiation.

Treatment of mice with hydroalcoholic extract of Tinospora cordifolia has been found to protect against the radiation-induced micronuclei formation and oxidative stress and decline in the mouse survival, spleen CFU and hematological parameters.

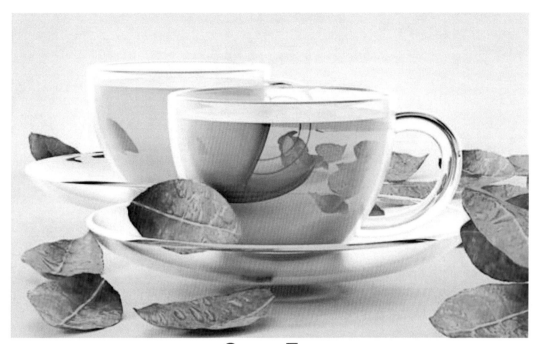

Green Tea

This is an antioxidant. Topical treatment containing green tea extract and the melatonin administration can prevent the cataract development. Topical treatment with green tea extract can be used to reduce the alpha particles effects on human skin because this polyphenol has antioxidant effects blocking the DNA methylation.

Internal use of antioxidants protects against cosmic radiation-induced oxidative stress.

Stepien et al. studied the effects of green tea extract oral administration in NaCl-induced hypertensive rats and observed, in serum, significant decreases of LDL and total cholesterol, molecules that can be the sources for reactive species synthesis in CR exposure.

## Hawthorn

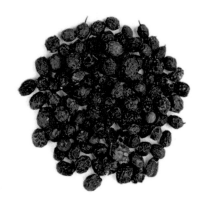

**Hawthorn has radioprotective properties against gamma irradiation in mouse bone marrow cells. Jan 01, 2007**

**Substances: Hawthorn**

**Diseases: Radiation-Induced Illness, Radiation-Induced Illness: Bone Marrow**

**Pharmacological Actions: Radioprotective**

**Additional Keywords: Plant Extracts**

## Heart-Leaved Moonseed, also known as, Guduchi, Guduchi, and giloy.

**Oral administration of an aqueous extract of Guduchi, Tinospora cordifolia has been reported to increase the survival of mice exposed to radiation. Treatment of mice with hydroalcoholic extract of Tinospora cordifolia has been found to protect against the radiation-induced micronuclei formation and oxidative stress and decline in the mouse survival, spleen CFU and hematological parameters.**

## Hesperidin

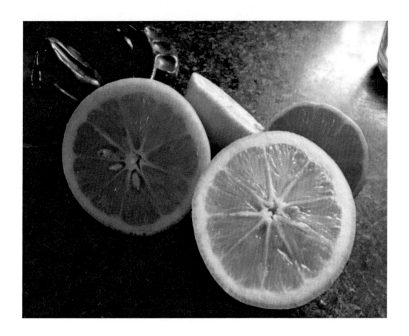

Hesperidin has a potential radioprotective agent against ionizing radiation-induced damage.Jul 11, 2019

Substances: Hesperidin

Diseases: Radiation

Pharmacological Actions: Radioprotective

Anti-Therapeutic Actions: Low Dose Ionizing Radiation

Hippophae rhamnoides, also known as, fruit juice concentrate

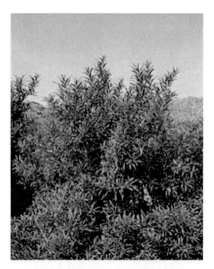

Common sea buckthorn shrub

*After three years of waiting, my Sea Berries should be fruiting next year. They are good to -50 degrees Fahrenheit. You need a male and female to fruit. This is known as Siberian Orange Juice. It has more anti-oxidant power than orange juice and no corn syrup*

When: Oral administration of a Hippophae rhamnoides fruit juice concentrate to rats before or after irradiation increased life span, restored the 11-oxycorticosteroid level in the blood and weight of isolated adrenals, and normalized their basal activity and response to (ACTH) (corticotropin) under in vitro conditions.

Hydroalcoholic extract of berries of H. rhamnoides also protected mice against γradiation-induced mortality, decline in endogenous colony-forming unit (CFU), micronuclei formation and various other hematological parameters.

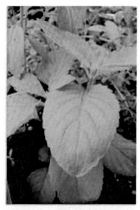
Close-up of *tulsi* leaves

## Ocimum sanctum, also known as, Holy Basil

*I was closing in for the harvest when the deer, AKA Brown Menace, jumped the fence and ate all the leaves down to the stem. Do they know something that we do not?*

Ocimum sanctum L. belongs to family Labiatae, commonly known as holy basil, tulsi or tulasi. Whole-plant extract contains flavonoids, alkaloids, saponins, phenols, anthocyanins, triterpenoids and tannins. Leaf extract contains flavonoids, alkaloids, saponins, tannins, phenols, anthocyanins, terpenoids and sterols.

The radioprotective activity of extract of O. sanctum was evaluated in mice through chromosomal aberration analysis.

When: The treatment of mice with extract of O. sanctum before irradiation resulted in faster recovery and reduced percentage of chromosomal aberrations in bone marrow cells. It was demonstrated that extract of O. sanctum offered in vivo protection against radiation-induced chromosomal damage and suggested that free radical scavenging could be the probable mechanism action.

Honey

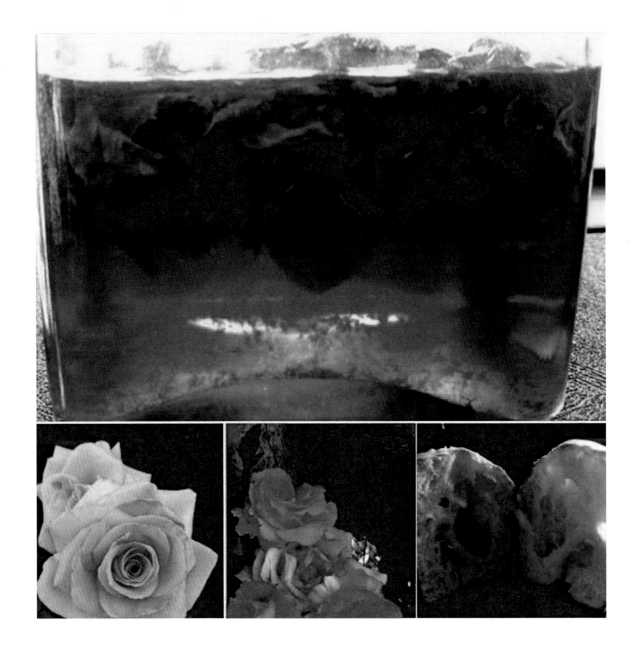

*I infuse my honey with many different things, including rose blossoms, culinary lavender, and lilacs. If you come visiting, warning, I also infuse hot peppers!*

Conventional honey is likely to be useful in the prevention and treatment of radiation- and chemoradiation-induced oral mucositis. Jan 31, 2019

Substances: Honey

Diseases: Radiation-Induced Illness: Mucositis

Pharmacological Actions: Radioprotective

# Kale and other cruciferous vegetables

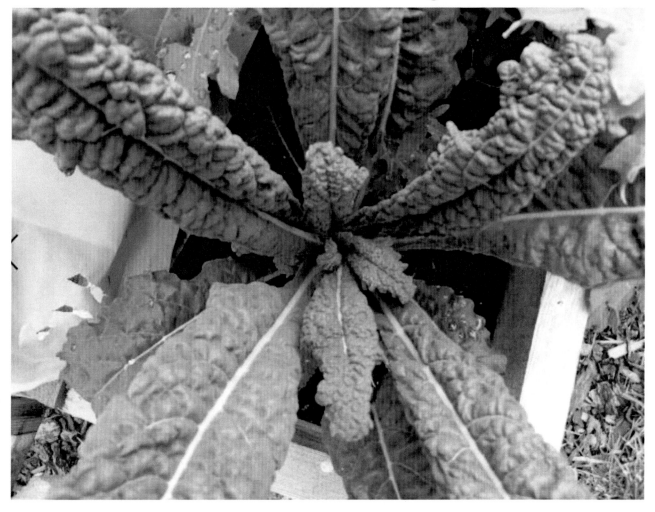

*Walk with the dinosaurs, Dino Kale, that is! Easy to grow and very tasty with that gnarly texture*

The radioprotective effects of sulforaphane, an Nrf2 inducer identified in cruciferous vegetables (broccoli, Brussels sprouts, cabbages), were studied by Mathew et al. on human skin fibroblasts.

The study showed that sulforaphane has dose-dependent effects and may protect against ionizing radiation damages if it is administered repeatedly before the fibroblast exposure.

# Lavandula angustifolia, also known as, English Lavender (use

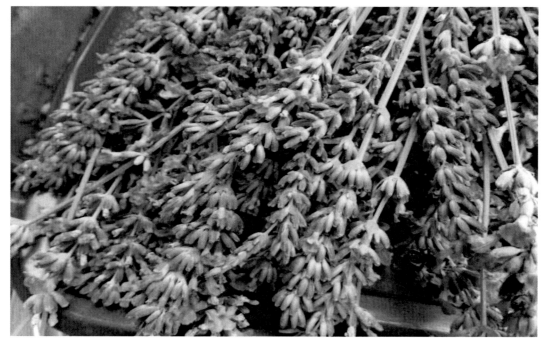

## Culinary Lavender)

*I use lots of lavender. Delight your family with a cream cheese with culinary lavender and a bit of honey on crackers. After blending refrigerate for about an hour for best results! Only use culinary lavender because other lavender has a toxin, which is alright for topical use but not consumption.*

**Lavandula angustifolia belongs to the family Lamiaceae. A total of 47 compounds representing 98.4–99.7% of the oils were identified. 1,5-dimethyl-1-vinyl-4-hexenyl butyrate was the main constituent of essential oil (43.73%), followed by 1,3,7-octatriene, 3,7-dimethyl- (25.10%), eucalyptol (7.32%) and camphor (3.79%).**

**Lavandula angustifolia oil was assessed for its radioprotective activity against UV radiation and γ-irradiation. EPR spectroscopy and UV- and γ-irradiated oil samples have shown excellent DPPH radical scavenging activity.**

It was suggested that after appropriate UV- or γ-irradiation treatment, lavender oil may have use as radioprotector and antioxidant for possible application in cosmetic and pharmaceutical industry.

**NOTATION: If used internally, use culinary lavender. All lavender is acceptable for topical application.**

## Cymbopogon citrates, also known as, Lemongrass

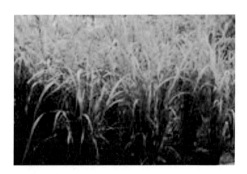

Cymbopogon citratus (family Poaceae), commonly called lemongrass. The chemical composition of the essential oil of C. citratus consists of compounds such as hydrocarbon terpenes, alcohols, ketones, esters and aldehydes. The essential oil is mainly composed of citral, which is a mixture of two stereoisomeric monoterpene aldehydes, the trans-isomer geranial and cis-isomer neral. It has been reported to contain flavonoids and phenolic compounds such as luteolin, quercetin, kaempferol and apigenin. Glycosyl derivatives of the flavones apigenin and luteolin have been identified in infusions of the lemongrass leaves.

Aqueous extract of C. citratus showed antioxidant and radioprotective properties. The extract was effective in reducing lipid peroxidation in irradiation and able to scavenge DPPH and superoxide radicals at low concentrations and protect DNA damage induced by radiation in pBR322 plasmid.

# Lichens

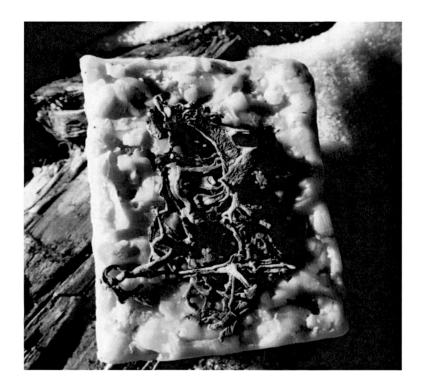

*This is Oakmoss, a lichen, adorning the top of one of my DIY goat milk soaps. Check out the anti-viral potential of lichens, you will be impressed!*

**High altitude saxicolous lichens can be an interesting source of new antioxidative substrates.Dec 31, 2013**

**Substances: Lichens**

**Diseases: Cancers: All, Oxidative Stress**

**Pharmacological Actions: Antioxidants, Cytotoxic, Radioprotective**

**Additional Keywords: Plant Extracts**

# Nigella sativa, also known as, Love in the Mist or Black Seed

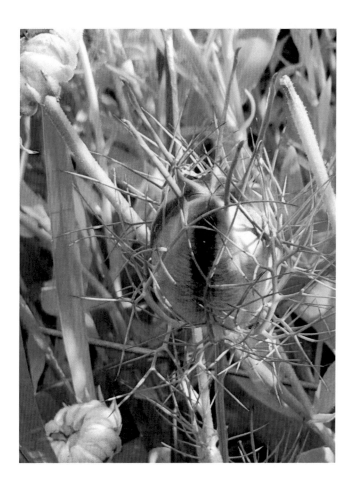

**Nigella sativa belongs to the family Ranunculaceae and is commonly called black seed. The most important active compounds of black seeds are thymoquinone, thymohydroquinone, dithymoquinone, p-cymene, carvacrol, 4-terpineol, t-anethol, sesquiterpene longifolene α-pinene and thymol, among**

**others. Seeds also contain alkaloids as isoquinoline and pyrazole ring bearing alkaloids. The extract of N. Sativa was evaluated in mice to assess protection against radiation-induced damage. Nigella sativa extract treatment showed significant reduction in lipid peroxidation and intracellular reactive oxygen species in splenocytes and increased the survival rate of irradiated animals, suggesting a radioprotective potential of N. Sativa.**

**When: Oral administration of N. Sativa oil before irradiation resulted in significant increase in blood malondialdehyde, nitrate and nitrite levels and antioxidant enzymes.**

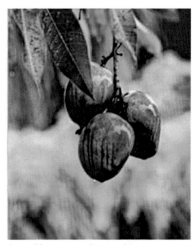

Mangifera indica, also known as, Mango

Mangifera indica belongs to the family Anacardiaceae and is commonly called mango or aam in Hindi. It has potent antioxidant, anti-lipid peroxidation, immunomodulation, cardiotonic, hypotensive, wound healing, antidegenerative and antidiabetic activities that are pharmacologically and medicinally important. It contains chemical contents such mangiferin, a polyphenolic antioxidant and a glucosyl xanthone. The bark is reported to contain protocatechuic acid, catechin, mangiferin, alanine, glycine, γ-aminobutyric acid, kinic acid, shikimic acid and the tetracyclic triterpenoids cycloart-24-en-3β26diol, 3-ketodammar-24 (E)-en-20S,26-diol, C-24 epimers of cycloart-25 en 3β24, 27-triol and cycloartenol-3β24,27-triol.

USE Notation: Use lower doses. The extract M. indica was evaluated for radioprotection in human lymphocytes and lymphoblastoid cells. Interestingly, it was noticed that that higher doses induced DNA damage in human lymphocytes and lymphoblastoid cells, without affecting the DNA repairability. However, protection was observed against radiation-induced DNA damage at lower doses of M. indica extract.

Pharmacological Actions: Anti-Allergic Agents, Anti-Inflammatory Agents, Antidiarrheals, Antifungal Agents, Antilipolytic, Antimalarials, Antioxidants, Antiparasitic Agents, Antiviral Agents, Immunomodulatory, Radioprotective

# Marigold

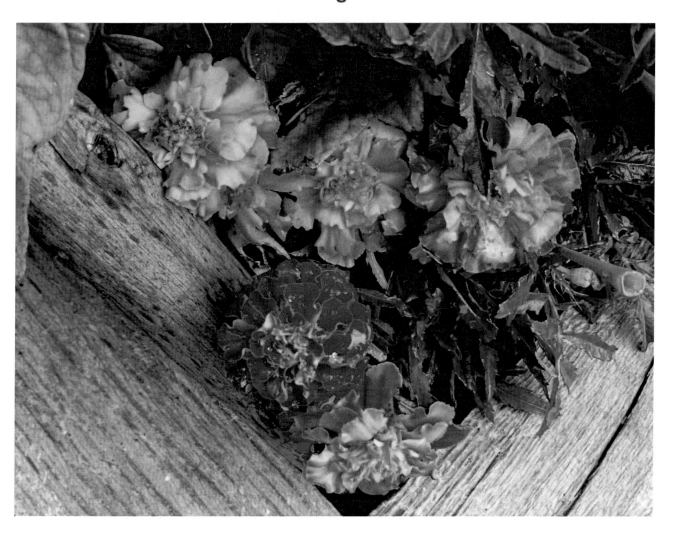

*Marigolds are a gardener's best friend because they keep the dreaded cabbage butterfly away! They also add color to your garden and are very easy to grow!*

This literature review discusses the topical agents studied for the treatment of acute radiation dermatitis. Feb 21, 2019

Substances: Aloe Vera, Catechin, Chamomile, Marigold, Vitamin C, Diseases: Chemotherapy and Radiation Toxicity, Dermatitis, Pharmacological Actions: Radioprotective

May Apple

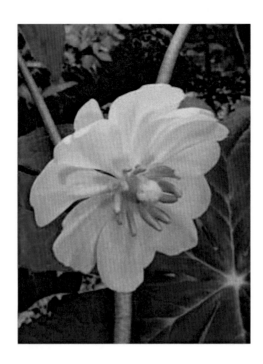

*I use this essential oil in my goat milk soaps. It has a rugged outdoors aroma.*

Podophyllum. hexandrum has been reported to protect against radiation-induced mortality, gastrointestinal damage, and embryonic nervous system of developing mice.

It has also been reported to protect against radiation-induced decline in glutathione-S-transferase, superoxide dismutase in the liver and intestine of irradiated mice.

## Heart-Leaved Moonseed, also known as, Guduchi, Guduchi, and giloy

Oral administration of an aqueous extract of Guduchi, Tinospora cordifolia has been reported to increase the survival of mice exposed to radiation. Treatment of mice with hydroalcoholic extract has been found to protect against the radiation-induced micronuclei formation and oxidative stress and decline in the mouse survival, spleen CFU and hematological parameters.

## Silymarin, also known as, Milk Thistle

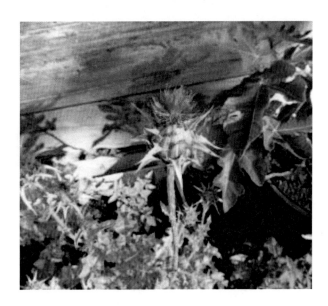

*Use organza bags over your thistle-heads to collect the thistledown when they "pop." Many thistles can be used to coagulate milk for cheesemaking for those who prefer an animal-free rennet*

**Beta-glucan and silymarin may protect against depleted uranium associated toxicity. Mar 01, 2011**

**Substances: Beta-glucan, Silymarin**

**Diseases: Uranium Poisoning**

**Pharmacological Actions: Radioprotective**

# Mentha arvensis, also known as, Mint

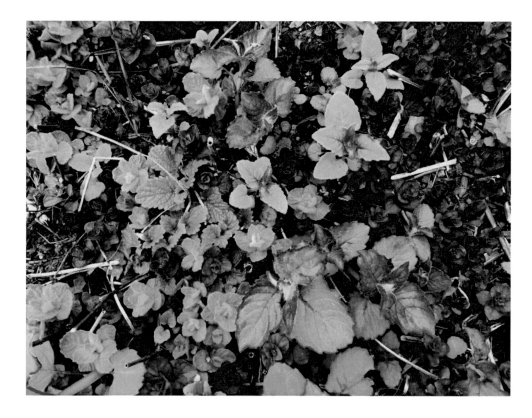

Dosage: Treatment of mice with 10 mg/kg b. wt. of chloroform extract of mint (Mentha arvensis Linn) protected against the radiation-induced sickness, gastrointestinal and bone marrow deaths with a DRF of 1.2. Further, it was non-toxic up to a dose of 1000 mg/kg b. wt., the highest drug dose that could be tested for acute toxicity.

When: Pre-treatment of mice with leaf extract of another species of pudina, i.e., Mentha piperita, has been reported to protect mice against the radiation-induced decline in hematological constituents, serum phosphatase, endogenous spleen colonies formation, spleen weight, goblet cells/villus section, and chromosomal damage.

Mint has radioprotective properties. Jul 01, 2010

Substances: Mentha Arvensis, Peppermint

Diseases: Radiation-Induced Illness

Pharmacological Actions: Radioprotective

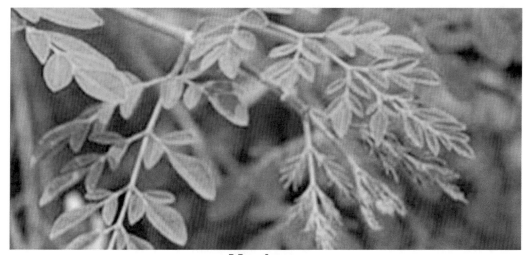

Moringa

A review of the biological activities of moringa oleifera leaves, seeds, bark, roots, sap, and flowers. May 31, 2015

Pharmacological Actions: Analgesics, Anti-Ulcer Agents, Antihypertensive Agents, Antioxidants, Cardioprotective, Hepatoprotective, Hypoglycemic Agents, Immunomodulatory, Radioprotective, Renoprotective

Myristica fragrance, also known as, Nutmeg

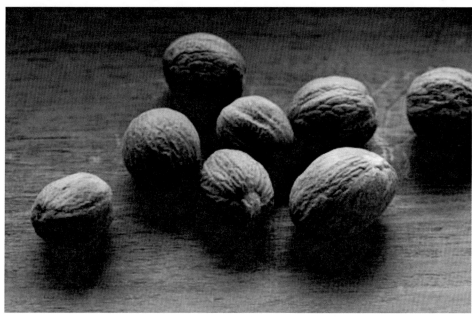

*Nutmeg is one of those versatile spices that you can use in cooking as well as health care products. I would like to grow a tree, but they get large, and it takes time for them to set fruit. Be careful with nutmeg, too much can produce hallucinations!*

Myristica fragrance belonging to family Myristicaceae is commonly called nutmeg and known for its antifungal, hepatoprotective and antioxidant properties. The chemical constituents include myristicin, lignan and eugenol. The essential oil of nutmeg contains mainly sabinene (15–50%), α-pinene (10–22%) and β-pinene (7–18%), with myrcene (0.7–3%), 1,8-cineole (1.5–3.5%), myristicin (0.5–13.5%), limonene (2.7–4.1%), safrole (0.1–3.2%) and terpinen4-of (0–11%).

Seed extract of M. fragrance was investigated for radioprotective effects in mice; it produced a dose reduction factor of 1.3.

When: Pretreatment of M. fragrance seed extract was effective in increasing the GSH content in liver and reduction of testicular lipid peroxidation level in mice. It was demonstrated that M. fragrance seed extract offers a great degree of radioprotection in terms of radiation-induced biochemical alterations and enhanced survival rate, suggesting its possible utility as radioprotector.

# Nigella sativa, also known as, Love in the Mist or Black Seed

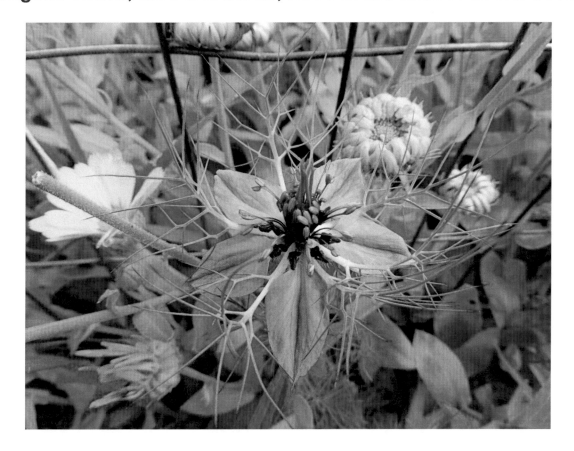

*Remember, it is the black seeds that hold the secret to health*

Nigella sativa belongs to the family Ranunculaceae and is commonly called black seed. The most important active compounds of black seeds are thymoquinone, thymohydroquinone, dithymoquinone, p-cymene, carvacrol, 4-terpineol, t-anethol, sesquiterpene longifolene α-pinene and thymol among others. Seeds also contain alkaloids as isoquinoline and pyrazole ring bearing alkaloids. Additionally, N. Sativa seeds contain α-hederin, a water-soluble pentacyclic triterpene and saponin.

Radioprotection by N. sativa extract and oil was studied in mice and rats. The extract of N. Sativa was evaluated in mice to assess protection against radiation-induced damage. Nigella sativa extract treatment showed significant reduction in lipid peroxidation and intracellular reactive oxygen species in splenocytes and increased the survival rate of irradiated animals, suggesting a radioprotective potential of N. Sativa.

**When: Oral administration of N. Sativa oil before irradiation resulted in significant increase in blood malondialdehyde, nitrate and nitrite levels and antioxidant enzymes.**

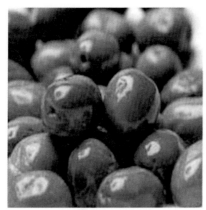

Olives

*I have not tried to grow olive trees here, but they do in Washington State, so maybe, I will give it a try.*

**Study demonstrated that in mice exposed to X-radiation that Olea europaea L. leaves extract is a potent radioprotective due to its mixture of polyphenols.**

# Allium cepa, also known as, Onion

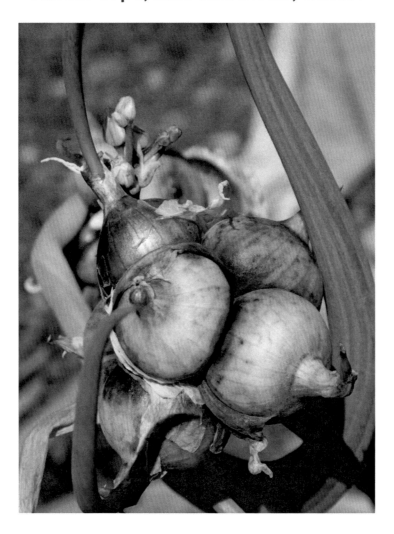

*How much fun is this? An onion with a top-notch of baby onions to plant for next year's onion crop!*

Allium cepa, belonging to the family Liliaceae that occurs worldwide, is a bulbous plant. Traditionally, it is used for the treatment of stomachache, throat infection and hepatitis, and has properties such as antioxidant, antihyperglycemic, antihypertensive and anti-asthmatic. Among the many photo-active constituents documented, the essential oil of A. cepa contains compounds such as 3-1,8-cineole, L-linalool and camphordare and has been thoroughly investigated. Besides this, the onion bulb contains Kaempferol, β-sitosterol, ferulic acid, muriatic acid and prostaglandins. Flavonoids and tannins are also present in A. cepa. Quercetin, quercetin 4-glucoside, taxifolin, taxifolin 7-glucoside and phenylalanine have been isolated from the bulb. The major sulfur compounds are dimethyl trisulfide, propenyl propyl disulfide, dipropyl disulfide, propenyl-methyl disulfide and methyl propyl trisulfide dipropyl trisulfide. Onion contains active compounds such as allyl propyl disulfide along with other active sulfur-containing compounds.

Radiation protection and antioxidative effects of onion extract were studied in albino rats. Biochemical parameters were assessed such as alanine aminotransferase, superoxide dismutase and catalase in liver, kidney, and heart. It was concluded that onion extract has significant radioprotective activity.

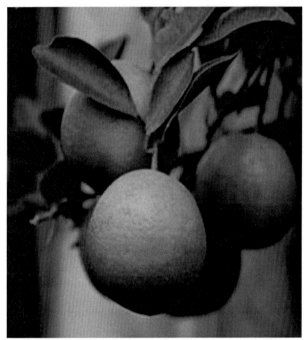

Citrus aurantium, also known as, Bitter Orange

*A favorite in Persia! Did you know that Iran has the most diversity and quantity of radio-protective plants of all the countries in the world?*

A favorite in Pdersiaitrus aurantium. The essential oil of Bitter Orange possesses antianxiety and motor relaxant effects in rats and mice. The main flavonoids occurring in cultivated citrus species are flavanone glycosides, hesperidin and naringin, accounting for 5% of dry weight of leaves and fruits. These exhibit vigorous antioxidant activity.

Dose: Citrus extract at different doses (250, 500, and 1000 mg/kg) have shown radioprotective effects against 1.5 Gy γ-irradiation in mouse bone marrow; however, 250 mg/kg dose was found to be the optimum dose, providing 2.2-fold protection. Radioprotective activity was assigned to the flavonoids contained in citrus extract.

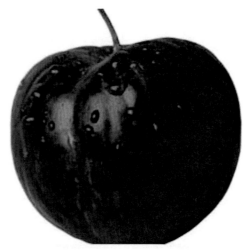

Syzygium cumini, also known as, Black Plum or Skeels

*Try a Black Plum Cake! It is very delicious and one slice is not enough*

Syzygium cumini - Skeels also known as Eugenia cumini (family Myrtaceae), and has been reported to possess several medicinal properties in the folklore system of medicine. The micronucleus study of radioprotective effect of dichloromethane and methanol (1:1) extract of jamun (SCE) in human peripheral blood lymphocytes (HPBLs).

Dosage: Radioprotective potential, where 12.5 µg/ml SCE was found to reduce the micronuclei up to a maximum extent. In vivo evaluation further established its radioprotective activity where it was found to reduce radiation-induced sickness, gastrointestinal, and bone marrow deaths.

Not only leaf but the hydroalcoholic extract of jamun seeds (JSE) also exhibited a greatest protective effect at 80 mg/kg JSE. The JSE was more effective when administered through the intraperitoneal route at equimolar doses than the oral. The JSE treatment protected mice against the gastrointestinal as well as bone marrow deaths with a DRF of 1.24.

# Citrus Extract

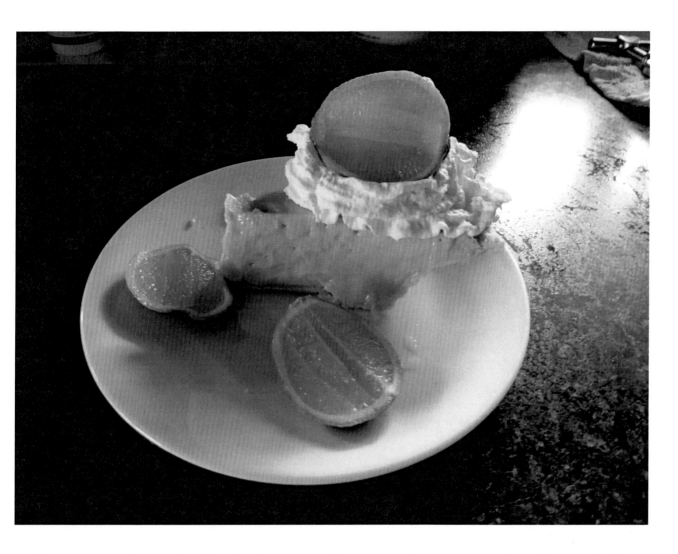

*I love my radio-protective in the form of my own home-grown key limes, in the form of Key Lime Pie. Radioprotection comes in many different forms!*

Dose:  At different doses (250, 500, and 1000 mg/kg) have shown radioprotective effects against 1.5 Gy γ-irradiation in mouse bone marrow; however, 250 mg/kg dose was found to be the optimum dose, providing 2.2-fold protection.

These exhibit intense antioxidant activity. Citrus extract at different doses (250, 500 and 1000 mg/kg) have shown radioprotective effects against 1.5 Gy γ-irradiation in mouse bone marrow; however, 250 mg/kg dose was found to be the optimum dose, providing 2.2-fold protection. Radioprotective activity was assigned to the flavonoids contained in citrus extract.

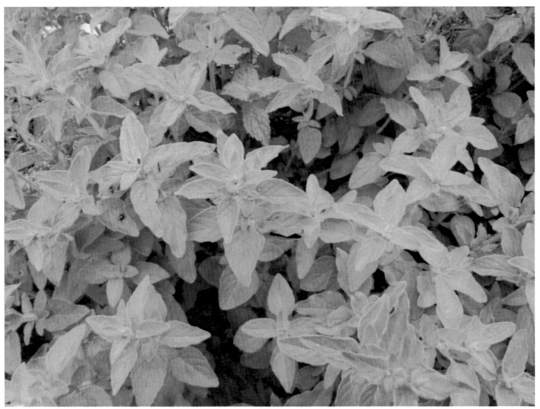

Origanum vulgare L., also known as, Oregano

*I have my hardy Oregano in my Italian raised bed. My favorite oregano recipe is Chicken Knickerbocker. A rice pilaf with chicken and pimentos with a generous drizzle or melted cheeses, spiced with oregano and nutmeg. Mouth-watering. That is tomorrow's dinner!*

Origanum vulgare belongs to the family Labiatae and is generally found as a wild plant in Europe and Iran. It is used for treating rheumatism, muscle and joint pain, sore and swellings as an external applicant. Oregano oil is employed to counter toothache. Antioxidants present in Oregano are rosmarinic acid, caffeic acid, flavonoids and derivatives of phenolic acids and α-tocopherol. Also, rosmarinic acid methyl ester, oregano-A and oregano-B act as antioxidants.

Radioprotection by Oregano extract was studied in terms of internal irradiation – as well as external irradiation-induced genotoxicity in human lymphocytes and mouse bone marrow. The oregano extract treatment resulted in significant reduction of micronuclei frequencies in human lymphocytes and mouse bone marrow. Radical scavenging activity of oregano extract was studied by DPPH assay, which shown that it was effective in scavenging of DPPH-free radical in dose-dependent manner. Therefore, free radical scavenging appears to be a likely mechanism for radioprotection.

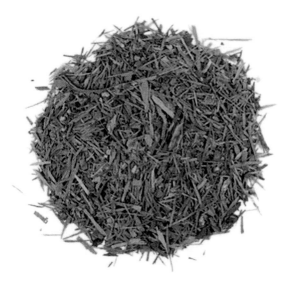

Pau d'arco

This is also called ipe roxo, la pacho, taheebo and bowstick tea) is an herbal tea from the inner bark of two trees that grow in the warmer part of South. Many South American doctors use a therapeutic tea from this herb to relieve pain and treat many conditions including leukemia and other forms of cancer, infections including yeast and other fungal diseases, skin rashes and many other ailments. Dr. Theodoro Meyer of the Universidad Nacional of Tucuman, a province of the Argentine Andes, studied taheebo's chemical composition and found a substance called xyloid, an antibiotic capable of killing viruses. Dr. Prats Ruiz, M.D., of Concepcion, a city in Tucuman province, reported blood profiles of patients with leukemia before and after treatment with taheebo to document the efficacy of taheebo in treatment of certain cancers. Clinical details are provided by Professor Carlos Hugo Burgstaller in his book on the medicinal flora of Paraguay and Argentina, La Vuelta a los Vegetales (Buenos Aires, 1968). This tea was widely available in many health food stores until news of its anticancer claims became widespread. There is now an FDA effort to prohibit its sale in the United States. It has already been taken off the Canadian market to be "reclassified as an over-the-counter drug" because of the healing claims made for it. FDA approval of a

**drug for a specific use takes 8-12 years and costs about $56 million (1982 estimate). It is radioprotective.**

# Pectin

**From 1996 to 2007, a total of more than 160,000 "Chernobyl" children received pectin food additives. As a result, levels of Cs-137 in children's organs decreased after each course of pectin additives by an average of 30-40%. Apr 01, 2009**

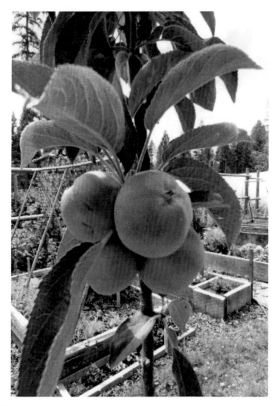

**Substances: Apple Pectin**

*Columnar apples in containers make it easy for garden enthusiasts who want radioprotection!*

**Diseases: Radiation Disaster Associated Toxicity, Radiation-Induced Illness: Cesium-137 Exposure**

**Pharmacological Actions: Detoxifier, Radioprotective**

# Capsicum annum, also known as, Hot Peppers

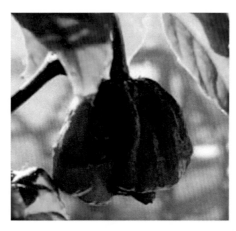

Capsicum annuum L. belongs to the genus Capsicum of family SolanaceaeCapsicum contains many chemicals, including water, fixed (fatty) oils, steam-volatile oil, carotenoids, capsaicinoids, resin, protein, fiber and mineral elements. Red peppers contain 280 µg/gm total carotenoids. Capsanthin accounts for 60% of the total carotenoids. They also provide 11% β-carotene and 20% capsorubin. Capsanthin is acylated with C12–18 saturated fatty acids.

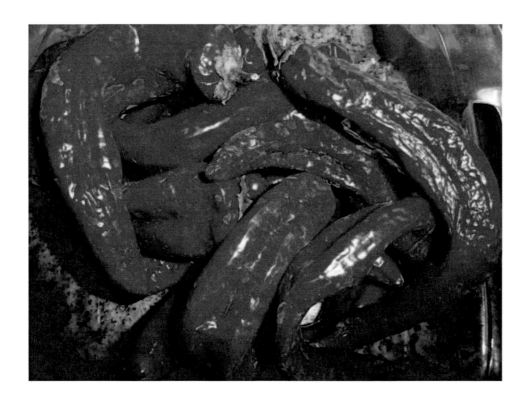

*On my farm, I grow 100 different kinds of peppers in all colors so I can eat the rainbow!*

The phenolic glycosides of C. annum L. were evaluated for their radioprotective effects, and oxidative damage induced by X-radiation was studied on human lymphocytes. Although these compounds showed less antiradical properties, they had higher radioprotective ability, and no cytotoxicity was observed.

## Mentha piperita, also known as, Peppermint

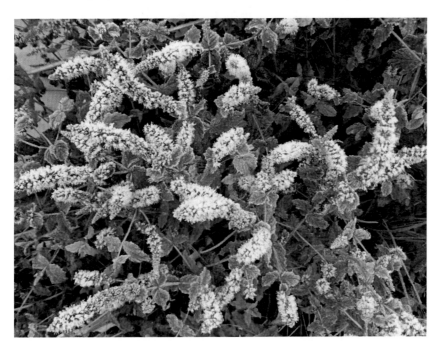

*Are you as smart as a Golden Retriever?  A guest had given me a Chocolate Mint, and my dog had an upset stomach, so she ate the plant.  LOL!*

Mentha piperita, commonly called peppermint, belongs to the family. It is an aromatic, stimulant and carminative and employed for treating nausea, flatulence and vomiting. Mentha extracts have antioxidant properties due to the presence of eugenol, caffeic acid, rosmarinic acid and α-tocopherol. Caffeic acid, rosmarinic acid, eriocitrin, luteolin-7-O-glucoside were identified as primary radical scavengers. It also contains phenolic acids, flavonoids, and s-carvone.

Mentha oil was found to afford radioprotection to hematological parameters and phosphatases level in mice. Treatment of M. Piperita extract prior exposure to γ radiation in mice has been shown to provide protection in bone marrow cells; it significantly reduced the number of aberrant cells and different chromosomal aberrations in irradiated mice.

**When: M. Piperita extract pretreatment was efficient in providing protection against hematopoietic injury in bone marrow, intestine and testis in mice.**

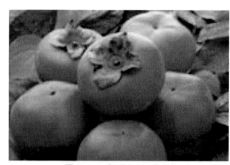
Persimmon

*My maternal grandmother had a persimmon tree. I did not care for the persimmons, but I enjoyed climbing the tree.  To be honest, I enjoyed the fall colored fruit too.*

**Extraction, purification, and anti-radiation activity of persimmon tannin.Sep 30, 2016**

**Substances: Persimmon**

**Diseases: Chemotherapy and Radiation Toxicity**

**Pharmacological Actions: Anti-Apoptotic, Radioprotective**

## Soybeans-Miso

**Made from naturally fermented non-GMO-soybeans, rice or barley, miso is an excellent source of usable whole protein, aids digestion, and assimilation is low in fats, has a nice salty flavor, promotes health and helps neutralize environmental pollution including radiation. The reason for Miso's protectiveness is not really known.**

**Miso was observed that the Japanese who ate miso every day did not die from radiation-induced cancer after the bombs at Hiroshima and Nagasaki. The observed effect of miso as a cancerostatic agent was further confirmed in a recent study in Japan.**

# Piper longum, also known as, Indian Long Pepper- family of black/white/red/green pepper

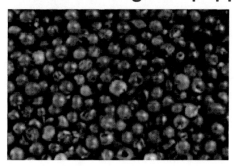

*This year I purpose to buy a pepper tree. I have fond memories of them from my youth. They do get large, but you can trim them. Radioprotection sealed the deal.*

Piper longum belongs to family Piperaceae. It is traditionally used as a medicine in Asia and the Pacific Islands for treating diseases such as gonorrhea, menstrual pain, tuberculosis, arthritis and is also used for analgesic, diuretic and muscle relaxant purposes. Chemical studies have shown that the genus Piper has many components including unsaturated amides, flavonoids, lignans, aristolactams, long and short-chain esters, terpenes, steroids, propenylphenols and alkaloids. The essential oils of ten Piperaceae species have shown that the most frequently identified compounds were sesquiterpenes. However, the nonoxygenated monoterpenes (Z) p-ocimene, a-pinene and b-pinene were prevalent as well. A biosynthetic approach showed that the most common sesquiterpenes identified, E-caryophyllene and germacrene D, have the E, E-farnesyl-PP as fundamental precursor and only two were originated from E, Z-farnesyl-PP reactions (a-copaene and d-cadinene).

The radioprotective effects of fruit extract of P. longum were studied in mice. Extract treatment prevented the radiation-induced depletion of white blood cells in mice. Extract treatment was also effective in declining the radiation-induced increased levels of glutathione pyruvate transaminase, alkaline phosphatase and lipid peroxidation thus offering protection to mice against radiation-induced damage. The ethanolic extract of Piper longum (pippali) fruits was found to protect mice against the radiation-induced decline in WBC, bone marrow cells α-esterase positive cells and GSH. Pippali extract also reduced the elevated levels of glutathione pyruvate transaminase (GPT), alkaline phosphatase (ALP), lipid peroxidation (LPO) in liver and serum of irradiated animals.

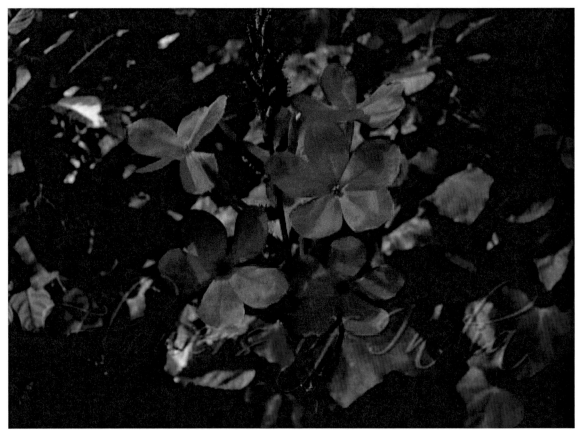

Plumbago Rosea, also known as, Rakta Chitrak

*Stunning flower!*

Plumbago Rosea L. belongs to the family Plumbaginaceae. It is variously used to treat diseases such as inflammation, skin diseases, gastric troubles and abdominal pain. It has active ingredients such as plumbagin, naphthoquinones, fatty alcohols, tannins and sitosterol glycosides. It has been reported that roots of P. Rosea contains several naphthoquinones and their derivatives and flavonoids. The chemical constituents include plumbagin, palmitic acid and myricyl palmitate from petrol extract, and plumbagin acid lactone, ayanin and azaleatin from ethyl acetate extract of roots.

The extract of P. Rosea was evaluated for antitumor activity. It has been reported that the P. Rosea extract possesses radiosensitizing effects and, combined with radiation, increases the tumor-killing effect.

# Potatoes, Sweet, Purple

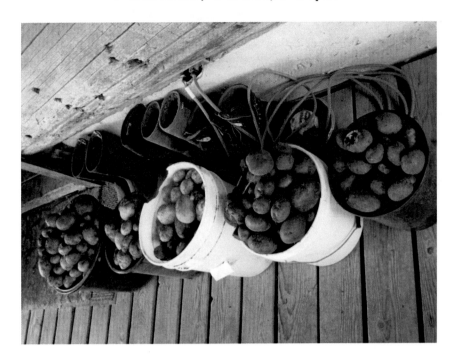

Abundant and so much fun to dig for potato treasure in the fall. My favorite potato recipe is Armenian Potatoes. Cut of potatoes, tomatoes, add minced garlic, ½ cup each of lemon juice and olive oil, a bit of water, salt to taste and lots of paprika. Parsley for a garnish!


Purple sweet potato pigments protective against Cobalt-60 induced radiotoxicity. Dec 01, 2010

Substances: Sweet Potato: Purple

Diseases: Radiation Associated Toxicity: Cobalt-60

Pharmacological Actions: Radioprotective

## Reishi

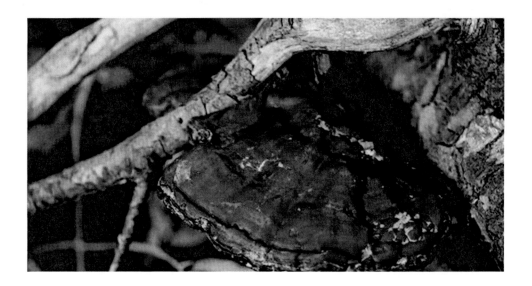

**Reishi extract protects against radiation and chemotherapy-associated toxicity.**
Oct 01, 2006

**Substances: Reishi Mushroom**

**Diseases: Chemotherapy-Induced Toxicity: Cisplatin, Liver Cancer, Radiation Disaster Associated Toxicity**

**Pharmacological Actions: Antiproliferative, Radioprotective**

## Resveratrol

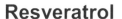

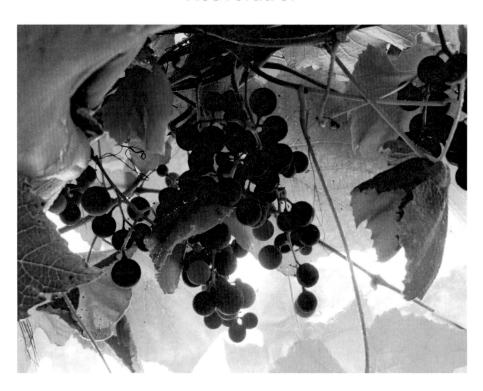

*Have your top canopy with grapes and your under-canopy herbs, peppers, or shade-loving flowers.*

Resveratrol (RSV), an natural polyphenol, is produced in several plants in response to injury, stress, bacteria or fungi infection, UV-irradiation and exposure to ozone. It is present in human diet i.e., in fruits and in wine. RSV is known for its antioxidant, anti-inflammatory, analgesic, antiviral, cardioprotective, neuroprotective and antiageing action and it has been shown to have chemopreventive effects concerning several human diseases such as cardiovascular disease, osteoporosis, and gastric ulcers. Depending on the dose, RSV may act as antioxidant or as pro-oxidant.

RSV improves sperm count and motility in rodents and prevents DNA damage caused by cryopreservation of human sperm. Moreover, RSV acting with other agents inhibits the toxic action of them. There are evidences that RSV can modulate the behavior of cells in response to radiation-induced damage. Minimalization of radiation-induced damage to somatic and germ cells by RSV might be useful in cancer therapy to prevent the damage to normal cells as well as in case of radiological accidents.

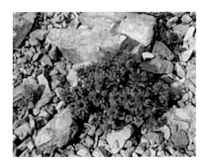
Rhodiola, also called, Kingy Herb

*Plants that must endure hostile environments to survive often have medicinal qualities to them.*

The roots have bioactive compounds to help cells produce energy. It is considered an adaptogen and helps remove toxins, radiation poisoning and addresses low oxygenation. When metabolism is increased, there is additional oxidative damage. Rhodiola protects from oxidative damage and helps the cell repair. Rhodiola has many attributes as it helps the heart, protects against radiation, enhances the chemotherapy effect for cancer, protects bone marrow and liver and gives more energy. It is essential to get a high-quality Rhodiola that is appropriately harvested and appropriately extracted.

The aqueous fraction exhibited significant ($P < 0.05$) pro-oxidant activity (up to 100 µg/ml) under metal ion-induced stress ± flux transition metal (Fe/Cu) ± 0.25 kGy.

Certain other active constituents involved in metal ion chelation contributed to the overall antioxidant activity. The methanolic fraction exhibited significant antioxidant activity up to 250 µg/ml, which contributed to its radioprotective efficacy. The aquo-methanolic fraction exhibited (disparate properties), i.e., concentration-dependent cytotoxicity (up to 250 µg/ml) and cytoprotection at 1000 µg/ml. R. imbricata, in general, exhibited a significant solvent-dependant variation in radioprotective efficacy.

IMPORTANT NOTE: Solvent extraction and dose are crucial in bioactivity modulation, and R. imbricata could be developed as a potential prophylactic radiation countermeasure for use in nuclear and radiological emergencies.

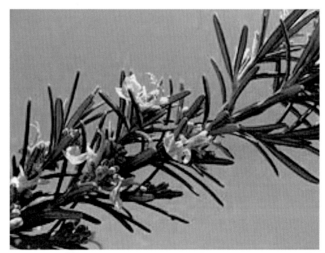

Rosmarinus officinalis, also known as, Rosemary

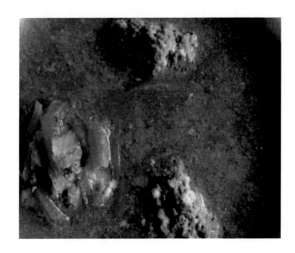

*Rosemary does great in drier climates and indoor cottage gardens if you live in the Rockies. I love my English Meat Dumpling and Rosemary Soup*

Rosmarinus officinalis L. belongs to family Labiatae. Rosemary leaves were found to have significant antioxidant properties and are extensively used in food industry due to its non-toxicity and safety. It contains antioxidants such as carnosic acid, carnosol, rosmarinic acid, rosmanol, isorosmanol and epirosmanol.

R. officinalis leaf extract was evaluated for its ability to protect the liver of mice against radiation-induced histopathological alterations. Extract treatment showed a significant decrease in lipid peroxidation and increase in GSH content in mice, and there was substantial decrease in binucleated hepatic cells as compared with untreated irradiated animals.

Rosemary has radioprotective and anti-mutagenic effects against chromosomal damage induced in human lymphocytes by gamma-rays. Mar 22, 2006

Substances: Rosemary

Diseases: DNA damage, Radiation-Induced Illness

Pharmacological Actions: Antimutagenic Agents, Radioprotective

# Rutin

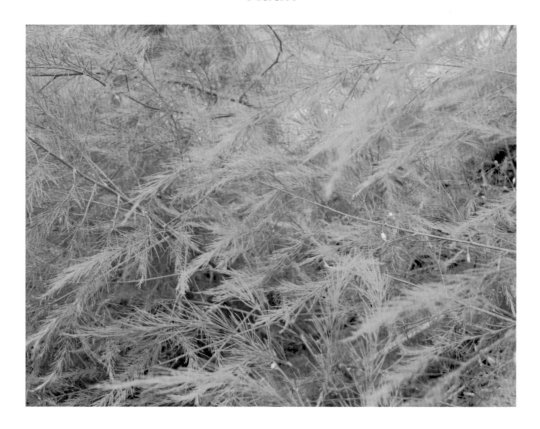

*Asparagus give you an opportunity to practice patience and companion planting*

Analysis of radioprotection and antimutagenic effects of Ilex paraguariensis infusion and its component rutin.Jul 15, 2018

Diseases: Chemotherapy and Radiation Toxicity

Pharmacological Actions: Antimutagenic Agents, Radioprotective

## Strawberries

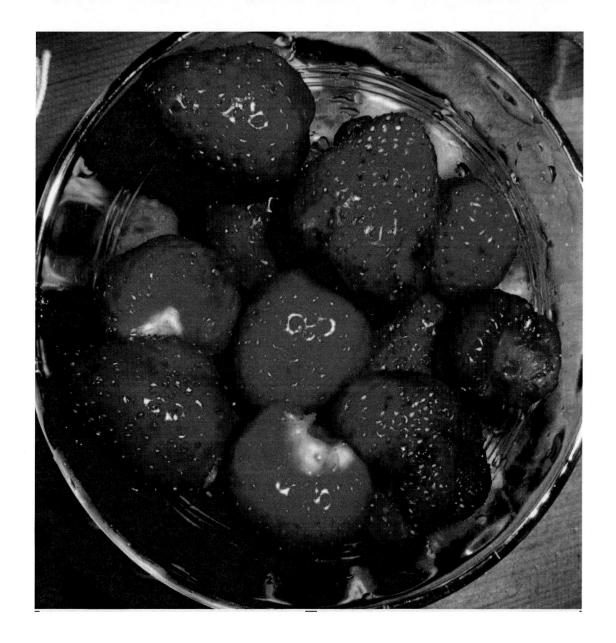

*Looks at these luscious strawberries. I had the PERFECT recipe picked out but the damn (sorry) choppers (chipmunks) ate them, gardening occupational hazard. Next year...*

Rabin et al. showed that strawberries can have a protective effect against the massive ion particles, and the dietary supplementation with these fruits can improve the protection against cosmic radiation.

## Saffron

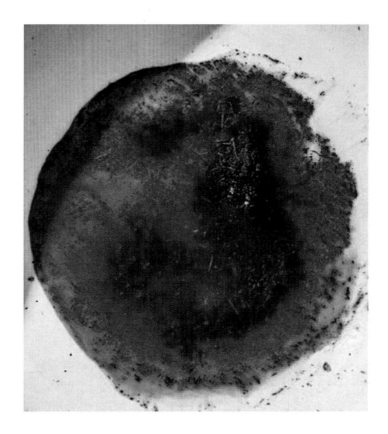

Koul and Abraham showed that saffron administration in mice inhibited the gamma-radiation induced oxidative stress and DNA damages. Crocin, picrocrocin and safranal are the active compounds of saffron. In a recent study, crocin and safranal prevented the DNA damages, and the testicular cells damages induced by the gamma-radiation and crocin also showed significant antioxidant effects, scavenging the hydroxyl radical.

Saffron tea. Saffron contains colchicine, a substance that has been used in the treatment of leukemia. It also lowers uric acid (high in those who have a tendency towards gout and/or cardiovascular disease).

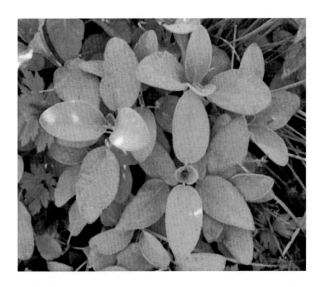

Salvia officinalis, also known as, Common Sage

*A leaf of sage a day preserves your memory as well as protects you from radiation. Good deal!*

Salvia officinalis belongs to the family Lamiaceae and is cultivated in several countries. It has remedial and household importance. The fragrance and aroma might be due volatile and essential oil that consists of mixture of volatile compounds such as terpenes, triterpenoids, ursolic acid and oleanolic acid. Antioxidants present are salvianolic acid (dimer of rosmarinic acid), carnosol, carnosic acid, rosmarinic acid, rosmanol, isorosmanol and epirosmanol.

The aqueous extract of S. officinalis showed significant radioprotection against irradiation in rats. Extract treatment resulted in decreased lipid peroxidation, protein carbonyl and NO in brain tissues and increased SOD and CAT enzymes activities and GSH contents. S. Officinalis extracts hold antimicrobial, anticancer, antioxidant, anti-inflammatory and radioprotective properties probably due to presence of active polyphenolic compounds that contains aromatic rings with hydroxyl groups.

Sesame seeds (raw)

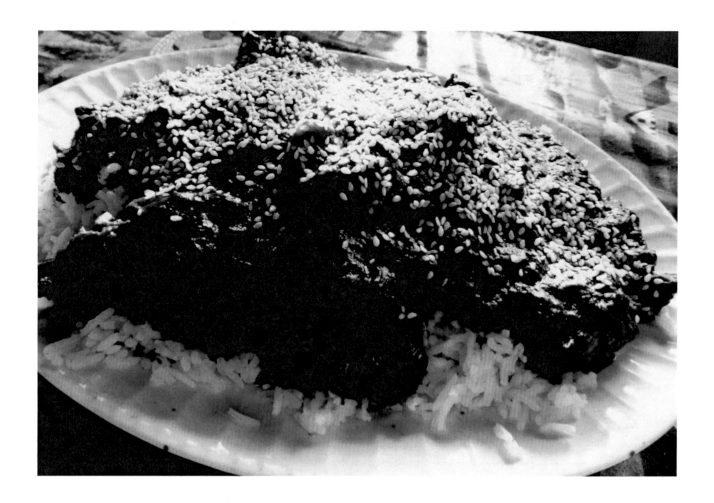

*Mole, mole-chocolate, nuts, fruit, 12 different peppers give a taste sensation to tantalize your taste buds. It is only hot if you choose to make it that way. Growing your own produce for Mole preserves indigenous recipes and pepper diversity.*

Sesame seeds – raw, ground (tahini) or in capsules. Sesame seed oil contains a substance called Complex T, the primary effect of which is to increase blood platelets - a must for fighting infection. In addition to Complex T, sesame seeds contain valuable essential fatty acids (EFAs) that are indispensable workers in the immune system.

Radioprotective and increases platelet level for anemic situations due to radiation.

Sesamol is a powerful radioprotective substance. Sep 07, 2011

Substances: Sesamol, Diseases: Radiation-Induced Illness,

Pharmacological Actions: Radioprotective

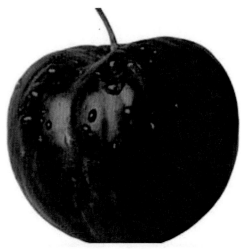

Syzygium cumini, also known as, Black Plum or Skeels

Skeels, also known as Eugenia cumini (family Myrtaceae), and has been reported to possess several medicinal properties in the folklore system of medicine.

The micronucleus study of radioprotective effect of dichloromethane and methanol (1:1) extract of jamun (SCE) in human peripheral blood lymphocytes (HPBLs) ascertained its radioprotective potential, where 12.5 µg/ml SCE was found to reduce the micronuclei up to a maximum extent. In vivo evaluation further established its radioprotective activity where it was found to reduce radiation-induced sickness, gastrointestinal, and bone marrow deaths. Not only leaf but the hydroalcoholic extract of jamun seeds (JSE) also exhibited a most excellent protective effect at 80 mg/kg JSE. The JSE was more effective when administered through the intraperitoneal route at equimolar doses than the oral. The JSE treatment protected mice against the gastrointestinal as well as bone marrow deaths with a DRF of 1.24.

## Soybeans-Miso

Made from naturally fermented non-GMO-soybeans, rice or barley, miso is a superior source of usable whole protein, aids digestion, and assimilation is low in fats, has a beautiful salty flavor, promotes health and helps neutralize environmental pollution including radiation. The reason for Miso's protectiveness is not really known.

Miso was observed that the Japanese who ate miso every day did not die from radiation-induced cancer after the bombs at Hiroshima and Nagasaki. The observed effect of miso as a cancerostatic agent was further confirmed in a recent study in Japan.

## Spirulina

**Spirulina has a radioprotective effect.**

**Substances: Spirulina**

**Diseases: Radiation-Induced Illness**

**Pharmacological Actions: Radioprotective**

## Illicium verum, also known as, Star Anise

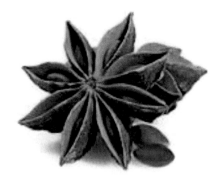

**Illicium verum, commonly known as Star Anise. The essential oil has confectionary application as a flavoring agent and industrial use in the preparation of Tamiflu to act against influenza virus. Anisyl acetone and benzene carboxylic acid were identified as the main phenolic components present in aqueous fraction of I. verum. I. verum extract showed radioprotective effects in irradiated minced chicken meat by reducing lipid peroxidation. It is an antioxidant.**

## Tea, Black

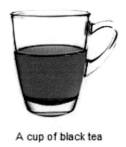

A cup of black tea

**Black tea extract protects against radiation-induced membrane damage of human erythrocytes. Oct 31, 2016**

**Substances: Black Tea**

**Diseases: Chemotherapy and Radiation Toxicity**

**Pharmacological Actions: Radioprotective**

## Ocimum sanctum, also known as, Tulsi Herb

**The radioprotective property of Ocimum sanctum was first reported by Jagetia et al. against the radiation-induced mortality, after that studies by Uma Devi and her coworkers established its radioprotective efficacy by evaluating mouse survival, spleen colony assay, and chromosome aberrations in mouse bone marrow cells. Apart from these osmium has been reported to protect against radiation-induced lipid peroxidation and reduction in glutathione concentration.**

## Curcuma longa, also known as, Turmeric

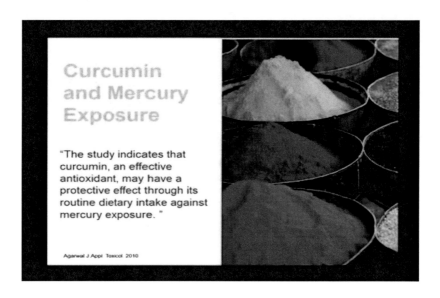

Curcumin and Mercury Exposure

"The study indicates that curcumin, an effective antioxidant, may have a protective effect through its routine dietary intake against mercury exposure."

Agarwal J Appl Toxicol 2010

*Turmeric is one of my top three herbs and easy to grow, even in the Rockies!*

Curcuma longa L. belonging to family Zingiberaceae. The chemical study of different samples of turmeric has yielded essential oil (4.2–14%), fatty oil (4.4–12.7%), and moisture (10–12.0%). It has been demonstrated that there are three major constituents curcumin, p-hydroxycinnamoyl (feruloyl)methane and p,p'-dihydroxydicinnamoylmethanel. Its oil has components such as sesquiterpene, ketones and alcohols.

Turmeric boosts immune system after CR exposure. Jelveh et al. established in their study that curcumin decreased the lipid peroxidation in fibroblasts membrane after gamma-irradiation.

When: Before and after irradiation

SYNERGY EFFECT: Turmeric and black pepper combined potentate both protections.

It has been suggested that there exist protective effects of curcumin against genetic damage as well as against the side-effects induced by 131I administration in terms of micronuclei frequency in human lymphocytes.

Radioprotective effects of C. longa extract were studied in rats against γ-irradiation, pre- and post-treatment. The extract was found to be effective in modulating the levels of inflammatory cytokines, trace elements, and the protein levels of SOD-1 and PRDX-1. Thus, modulation of antioxidant enzymes was held responsible for conferring radioprotection by C. longa extract.

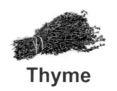

Thyme

**Thyme tea.**

**When: Used as a remedy after x-rays.**

**Dosage: One tablespoon of thyme per pint of hot water for 20 minutes, then cool and strain.**

## Valeriana wallichii, also known as, Valerian

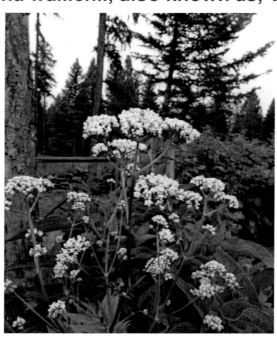

*Pretty plant but ones uses the roots.  Bees love it!*

**Valeriana wallichii, belonging to the family Valerianaceae. Its rhizome and root contains volatile oil (valerianic oil), which is composed of alkaloids, boryl isovalerianate, chatinine, formate, glucoside, isovalerenic acid, 1-camphene, 1-pinene, resins, terpineol, and valerianine. From compounds, such as citric acid, malic acid, maliol, succinic acid and tartaric acid, have been isolated.**

**When:** The root extract of V. wallichii was found to significantly protect against radiation-induced free radicals at 4 h after 5 Gy of irradiation,

**General** reduced prolonged oxidative stress led increase in mitochondrial mass, enhanced reproductive viability of cultured cells, and protected against radiation-induced DNA damage.

# Radio-Protective Foods in my Kitchen

# Radio-Protective Foods to Purchase

# Days of Awe!

As a proverbial adventurer and researcher, it is dreadfully painful to set boundaries, so that this book can get published. There are so many details and things left unsaid because the topic of health and nutrition is mostly a lost art these days. Besides, research is just emerging on the past 120 years of scientific data collect about radiation. Each day, there is more and more news coming to light. One prayer that I pray for each of you is that your encounter with eternal moments will not be accumulation of dying moments but that you will persevere with all joy that brings you to this season.

It is my prayer that you take this book to heart. We have but a short time to prepare ourselves for this extinction-level event. You must understand that it has already begun. 2019 is the Zeroth. This is Year 0, just as there is a Patient Zero for an epidemic or Ground Zero for a military action. We have all enjoyed years of abundance. From this year forward, we will gyrate into a cascading abyss of famines, wars, earthquakes, volcanism, and plagues. It is my firm belief that heaven has touched earth at pivotal times in history. With each act of kindness, love, steadfastness, and humanity, we impart light to the planet and to a broken mankind. It is my belief that we are entering the Days of Awe, where heaven touches earth, for one last cataclysmic epoch. Each of us has power within us to bring heaven to earth. And so, sky meets land where the divine presence shines unconcealed. This is the time and place where you can meet God.

You live in a unique time in history where the cycles of time are converging. The barriers between time, space, and dimensions are vanishing before our eyes. Creation itself has been replaced and we find ourselves in a war where the Laws of Nature that once protected and nurtured us. Like a magician's sleight of hand, all of the elements and forces of creation are no longer are our friends. They have become our adversaries. It is a calculated and scaled engagement from the Planck level (much smaller than atoms) to the furthest cosmos. The reality that we once knew and appreciated is gone forever. We are living in a new paradigm. This calls for a steep learning curve as the power elite have piggy-backed on to judgment of the Living God who is the Creator of All. As our protective barriers are removed, one by one, it will take time and effort for you to erect your own personal protective barriers. You have been given all the tools. Whether you choose to prepare physically, or spiritually, or both, it is imperative to begin of intensify your actions. This is your time of refuge.

May you use this energy of time for repentance, taking stock, breaking of damaging patterns, learning to be free, developing sensitivity, allowing yourself to be consoled and to console, allowing your tears to be caught in a bottle, and allow your broken heart to be healed.

Be of good cheer my friends! While the situation we find ourselves in is very dire, we have hope and confidence! Humanity has survived past extinction events, albeit this time, our survival may take a different form. These are eternal moments that will with a song in your heart lift you to an infinite time and place and the hardships which with we must endure in the next days as if it never was. Treasure these eternal moments because it will be at this time that your fleeting connection between infinite and finite will become one, forever. Focus on your destination, for you were born for such a time as this!

# Appendix 1

# Guide to Nutrition & Free Vitamins and Minerals

**Free Vitamins and Minerals**

**Did you know that the first vitamins were only discovered in 1913?**

**In the 1960's a list of food components and nutrients was completed including 50 substances and 22 types of amino acids (that form proteins) for nutrition.**

**Surprise! During the 1980's hundreds of plant-based components called phytonutrients were discovered through chemical analysis. A part is a chemical substance present in food:**

**• Natural as in the case of nutrients**

**• Accidental- as in the case of biological and chemical contaminants.**

**• Intentional-as with additives. Today biological and chemical contaminates are intentional.**

## Nutrients

**A nutrient is a food component that the body needs to carry out vital functions. Its chemical composition must be known. A food component is classified as a nutrient when its lack in the diet provokes a pathologic condition which disappears when the food component is again available to the body.**

**Most nutrition can be generated from consuming plants and animals, and the body takes it from there to make it bioavailable. There are a few substances that the body needs and it cannot generate so outside supplementation is necessary. Plant-based foods provide all nutrients except vitamin B12.**

**Classically: water, carbohydrates, proteins, fats, minerals, and vitamins are considered nutrients.**

**Carbohydrates your energy generators, and contribute to growth and repair and include proteins, fats, and minerals. Regulators intervene in various processes and functions of the body, and they contain vitamins, minerals, fiber, and phytochemicals.**

**Vitamins and minerals come in a shapes and sizes...just like us! There are pro's and con's for each option that you choose.**

**• Raw food a la natural has multiple advantages but is time-consuming to raise, collect, harvest and store. They are bio-available!**

• Fresh Food supplements contain many great health benefits but not quite as much as pure food. They are expensive but save you time. Bio-available!

• Mostly pure supplements and minerals are a high-end vitamin or mineral but has limited health function. Not as bioavailable.

• Half natural, half synthetic w/lots of adulterants have some specific targeted ingredients, but one misses the health advantage of layered raw food benefits

Totally artificial are toxic to the body. They are created in a lab and are more likely to kill you than enhance your health. They are cheap, and most are made in laboratories, primarily in China. Not bioavailable.

## Energy

Energy is defined as the capacity to perform work. It is not a component in food but rather the result of combustion of energy nutrients such as carbohydrates, fats, and proteins. NEWS Flash: Global government mandates reduced carbohydrates, fats and proteins. This produces obesity, growth retardation, and physical weakness. Energy is not lost during food processing. You need to increase energy nutrition during physical exercise and stressful situations.

Fact-Checker: Olive oil has the highest energy value and of animal nutrients, lard, and unsalted butter come in the highest.

## Proteins

Proteins are formed by the union of amino acids. There are essential and non-essential amino acids. Their function is to create and maintain your tissues, synthesize antibodies against infection, form blood hemoglobin, produce enzymes, and energy.

Deficiency of protein will cause weakness, apathy, immunodeficiency, edema, and liver failure.

Overly consumed protein causes renal and rheumatic diseases, gout, and acidification of blood.

Fact-Checker: The highest plant proteins are soy and lentils. The highest animal proteins are Gruyere cheese and canned tuna in oil.

Carbohydrates Carbohydrates can be simple or complex. They are the primary source of energy in our body.

**A deficiency of carbohydrates causes acidification of the body known as ketosis, mineral loss, dehydration, and consumption of protein.**

**Too much proteins causes malnutrition and dystrophy in children.**

# Fiber

**Fiber is the cellulose, hemicellulose, pectin, mucilage and other polysaccharides in plants. Fiber reduces constipation, diverticulosis, colon cancer, and hemorrhoids while protecting intestinal mucosa.**

**A deficiency of fiber can cause constipation, diverticulosis, colon cancer, and hemorrhoids.**

**Too much fiber can cause loss of absorption of iron, zinc, and other minerals and can irritate the intestines causing colitis.**

**Processing: Refined grains lose up to 95% of their fiber.**

**Fact-Checker: Bran and lentils have the highest fiber in plant-based foods while no animal product contains any fiber.**

# Vitamins

## Vitamin A

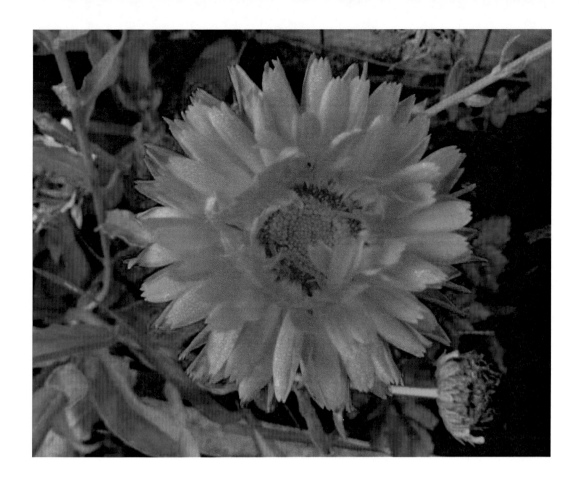

*Calendulas are beautiful, easy to grow, eatable, and dehydrate well.*

Vitamin A retinol and dehydroretinol found in animal foods, primarily liver and milk fat's and can be toxic. It used to be called the miracle vitamin because of its effect on the immune system

Provitamin A includes carotenes and beta-carotenes found in orange vegetables, carrots, peppers, and some dark greens such as spinach, and present no risk of toxicity.

Vitamin A is involved with numerous bodily processes, including vision, growth, bone and tooth development, skin, healthy mucosa, and protection against cancer. They also contain antioxidants that protect the heart and arteries. I personally find that Vitamin A supplementation during the first 5 days of any signs of infection quickly eliminates or reduces a viral or bacterial infection. Anti-Aging may help hyperthyroidism, improves night vision.

Let's go wild!

• Plaintain

- **Wild Strawberries**

- **Dandelion**

- **Water Cress**

- **Chickweed**

- **Elderberry Flower**

- **Lambs Quarters**

- **Purslane**

- **Nettles**

- **Rose Hips**

- **Into the garden:**

- **Calendula**

**Deficiency includes vision disorders, dry skin, fetal development disorders.**

**Processing: 15-35% of Vitamin A is lost in cooking. Sunlight, ultraviolet light, destroys vitamin A. Freezing does not impact Vitamin A.**

**Fact-Checker: Carrots and apricots have the highest plant-based Vitamin A. Beef liver and butter have the highest animal-based Vitamin A.**

Vitamin B1

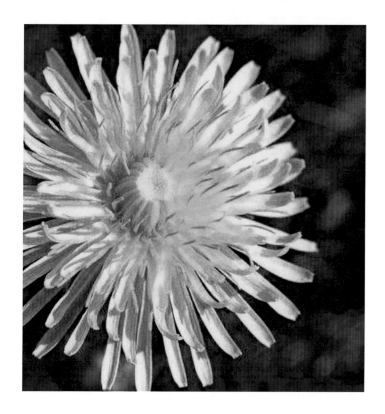

*Dandelions may be a weed, but they make an excellent blood tonic for the spring and also delicious fritters.*

**Vitamin B1 is also called thiamine.**

**Vitamin B1 is found in seeds, grains, and brewer's yeast. Animals have some traces of Vitamin B1 but it is tiny.**

**Let's go wild!**

**• Asparagus (Asparagus Officinalis)**

**• Fireweed**

**• Dandelion**

**• Elderberry Flower**

**• Red Clover**

**• Wild Amaranth**

**• Tea and poorly cooked fish and shellfish can destroy Vitamin B1.**

Thiamine is essential for the metabolism of carbohydrates and energy production. It is also necessary for the stability of the nervous system promoting mental and psychological health and wellbeing.

• May be useful in treating heart disease.

• May be beneficial in the treatment of neurological disease.

• May help treat anemia.

• May improve mental agility.

• May help control diabetes.

• Useful in treatment of herpes and infections.

Deficiency Symptoms: Nervous disorders, apathy, fatigue, irritability, depression, digestive disorders such as lack of appetite, slow digestion, and constipation, circulatory disorders like heart failure, and polynephritis inflammation of the peripheral nerves.

Increase: nervous disorders, nicotine addiction, drug addiction, alcoholism.

Processing: Bread baking causes a loss of 15-30% of Vitamin B1. Cooking vegetables net a loss of 25% and cooked meat or fishnets a loss of 30-50%.

Fact-Checker: Sunflower seeds and wheat germ have the highest plant-based thiamine while pork products have the highest animal-based, that said animal-based is minuscule.

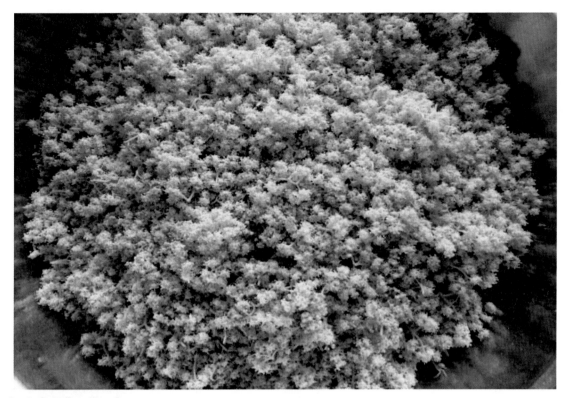

**What is it? Riboflavin**

*Elderberry flowers are a world-renown anti-viral. I make wine with them that tastes like pink grapefruit with floral notes. Delicious!*

**Where is it found? It is found abundantly in plant and animal origins.**

**What is its function? Riboflavin is necessary for all chemical reactions in which energy is processed in the body from carbohydrates, fats, and if the other two are exhausted animal protein. It forms the pigment in the retina (eye) and is necessary for vision. It is essential for the synthesis of corticoid hormones in the cortex of suprarenal glands. It prepares the body for stress.**

**Let's go wild!**

**• Elderberry Flower**

• **Nettles**

• **Wild Amaranth**

• **Dandelion**

• **Plantago**

• **Deficiency symptoms: Fatigue, weakness, apathy, vision disorders, dermatitis, skin eruptions, and anemia.**

**When to increase it: Stress, fatigue, vision disorders, dermatitis, skin eruptions, eczema.**

**Processing: Riboflavin is very heat tolerant but still looses between 10-20% during cooking. Dehydration and freezing has little effect.**

**Fact checker: Soybeans and bran are the highest plant-based sources while fresh egg yolks and cheese are the highest animal sources.**

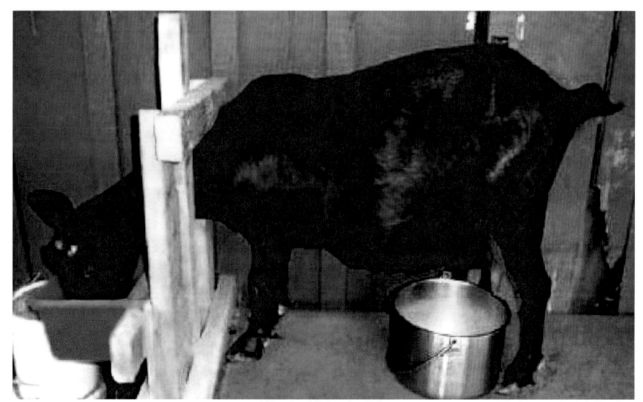
Niacin-Vitamin B3

**What is it?** It can be known as niacin, PP factor, or Vitamin B3. It has two active substances: nicotinic acid and nicotinamide (not to be confused with nicotine in cigarettes). It is found in milk, eggs, fish, and meat. It works with the amino acid Tryptophan.

**What is its function?** It intervenes as a coenzyme in energy production in the cells. It is necessary for body growth. Plant-based niacin reduces cholesterol levels.

**Deficiency symptoms:** Skin disorders, nervous system disorders, including depression and anxiety.

**Let's go wild!**

• **Elderberry Flower and Red Clover**

• **Wild Amaranth**

**When to increase it: Growth and pregnancy**

**Processing: Niacin is heat and light tolerant. There is little loss in processing or long term food storage.**

**Fact checker: Tuna in oil and animal livers are the highest source of niacin in animals while plant-based niacin is highest in bran and peanut butter and wheat germ.**

Vitamin B6

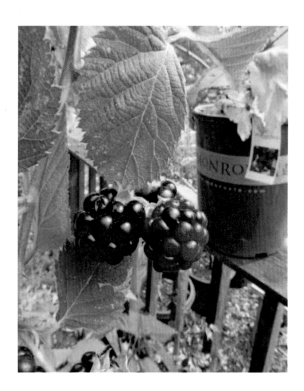

*I just found this Blackberry and Peony Homemade Ice Cream Recipe.  Yum!*

**What is it? Vitamin B 6 is pyridoxine, pyridoxal, pyridoxamine.**

**Where is it found? It is located in whole grains, legumes, some fruits such as bananas.**

**Let's go wild!**

**• Asparagus (Asparagus Officinalis)**

**• Wild Berries (black and blue)**

**What is its function?**

**• Metabolism of proteins. It facilitates the absorption of amino acids and their assimilation to body proteins.**

**• Metabolism of carbohydrates and fats, allowing these nutrients to be transformed into energy.**

**• Energy production within the cells of the nervous system.**

• Blood formation in involved in the synthesis of hemoglobin that forms red blood cells.

Deficiency symptoms: Fatigue, nervousness, anemia, skin disorders

When to increase it: If taking contraception, pregnant, nursing, TB, neuropsychological patients.

Processing:

Refined grains (includes bread and pasta): 75% loss

Refined sugar: 100% loss

Cooking: 25-50% loss

Canning: 40-50% loss

Fact checker: Salmon and beefsteak are the largest animal-based source with bran, wheat germ, and garlic being the top plant-based sources.

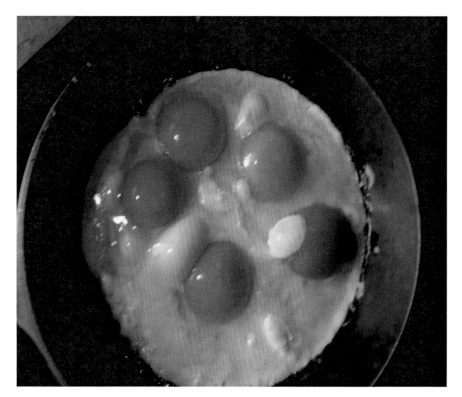

Vitamin B12

*Free-range chickens have orange yolks because customers want that. So....the commercial feed industry figured out a way to put a dye in chicken feed that turns the yolks orange. That is why you need to know your farmer or be your farmer.*

**What is it? Cyanocobalamin or variant**

**Where is it found? Higher animals do not produce this vitamin, but they store it in their liver. Milk and eggs and fish contain B12. Specific yeasts during fermentation can produce B12.**

**What is its function?**

**B12 is necessary for cell division, formation of red blood cells, and formation of myelin the fiber that protects the nerves.**

**Let's go wild!**

**• Wild Amaranth**

**• Wild Sea Buckthorn**

**Deficiency symptoms: Anemia and nervous disorders. I can attest that being low in B12 can impact cognition and energy also.**

**When to increase it: If you are a vegetarian.**

**Processing: Cooking destroys 30% of B12, pasteurization of milk about 10%**

**Fact checker: Beer and white bread are the highest sources of plant-based B12 while animal-based B12 is found in animal liver, caviar, fish and eggs.**

Folic Acid

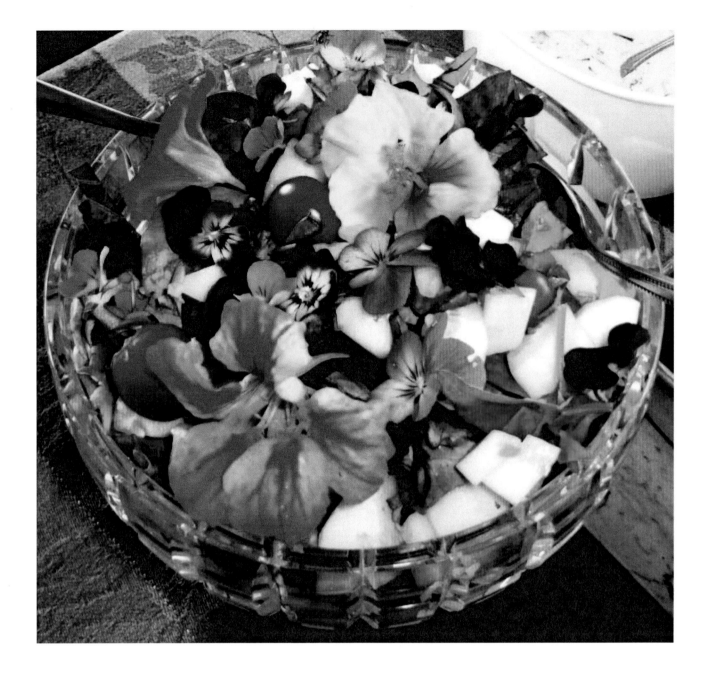

*Why can't salad be art?*

**Where is it found?** Legumes are a significant source followed by leafy greens and nuts. Milk, fish, and meat are low in folates.

**What is its function?** Folates are essential for the synthesis of DNA and RNA, which make up the basis of our life. It is involved with hemoglobin production and other physiological processes.

**Deficiency symptoms:** Anemia, glossitis (of the tongue), mental deterioration, congenital malformations of fetal nervous system.

When to increase it: Growth periods, pregnancy, cardiac disease, consumption of alcohol, cancer treatment, epileptic medications, and parasites.

Processing: Extremely unstable in light or heat.

Cooking and canning reduce folates: 50-95%

Storage of vegetables: 50-75% folate lost at room temperature.

Folates are not impacted by refrigeration.

Fact checker: Mung beans and chickpeas are the largest plant-based source of niacin while cheese and fresh eggs are the highest source for animal-based foods. That said, plant-based foods are significantly higher in niacin.

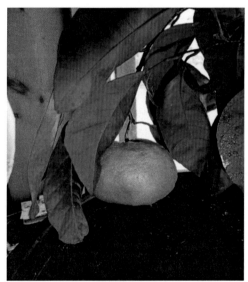
Vitamin C

*Imagine picking your own Mandarin Oranges from your windowsill orchard!*
What is it? Ascorbic acid.

Where is it found? Plants and most animals can synthesize it from glucose, but humans cannot, nor can they store it. They must take it daily!

What is its function?

It is an antioxidant that neutralizes free radicals, which cause cellular aging, DNA deterioration, and cancer.

• It is an antitoxin that neutralizes a variety of toxins, including those found in cured meat.

• It strengthens the immune system against infection.

• Contributes to collagen formation and is necessary for wound healing.

• Improves bones and teeth.

• Strengthens capillary and arterial walls.

• Facilitates absorption of nonheme iron.

Let's go wild!

• Asparagus

• Fire Weed

• Plantain

• Wild Strawberries

• Dandelion

• Dog rose (Rosa canina), fruit, 1252 mg

• Balsam fir (Abies balsamea), needles, 270 mg

• Eastern white pine (Pinus strobus), bark and needles, 200 mg and 32 mg respectively

• Garlic mustard (Alliaria petiolata), aerial parts, 190 mg

• Red spruce (Picea rubens), needles, 169 mg

• Wild garlic (Allium vineale), leaves, 130 mg

• Garden yellow-rocket (Barbarea vulgaris), basal leaves, 130 mg

• Common blue violet (Viola sororia), basal leaves, 130 mg

- Lamb's quarters (Chenopodium album), whole young plants, 130 mg

- Elderberry (Sambucus nigra), fruit, 116 mg

- Shepherd's purse (Capsella bursa-pastoris), basal leaves of first-year plants, 91 mg

- Wild leeks (Allium tricoccum), leaves, 80 mg

- Woodland strawberry (Fragaria vesca), fruit, 80 mg

- Mock strawberry (Duchesnea indica), leaves, 79 mg

- Eastern redbud (Cercis canadensis), flowers, 69 mg

- Mountain ash (Sorbus aucuparia), fruit, 68 mg

- Common yellow woodsorrel (Oxalis stricta), leaves, 59 mg

- Northern white cedar (Thuja occidentalis), needles, 45 mg

- Curley Dock

- Pine Needles replenish your vitamin C levels – pine needle tea had 3 – 5 times as much vitamin C as orange juice.

Deficiency symptoms: Fatigue, poor wound healing, bleeding, scurvy

When to increase it: Nicotine addiction, stress, infection, wound, burns

Processing: Vitamin C is the most sensitive of all vitamins. Heat, light, dehydration destroys 75% of this Vitamin C.

Fact checker: Beef liver, oyster, trout are the highest animal-based source of Vitamin C while Red Sweet Peppers, Guava, and Black currants are the highest plant-based Vitamin C sources. Rose hips can be used for high vitamin C but they must be used fresh or they lose their Vitamin C.

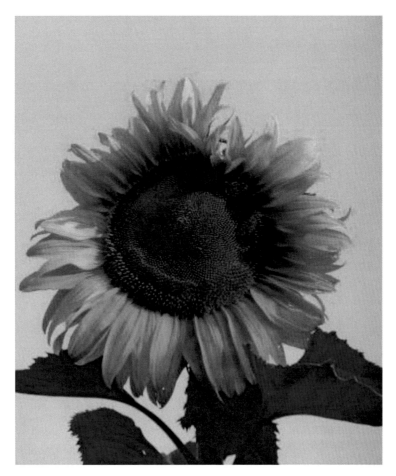

Vitamin E

***Mammoth Siberian Sunflower provides enough seeds for planting, eating, and feeding the wildlife***

**What is it? It is also known as tocopherol**

**Where is it found? It is found in grain germ, particularly wheat, sunflower seeds, nuts, olives, avocado.**

**What is its function?**

**Vitamin E protects the integrity of the cells and prolongs their life span.**

**• It is an antioxidant that prevents oxidation of vegetable oils.**

**• Neutralizes harmful free radicals from chemical contamination and body activity within cell walls.**

• Protective action against cancer and arteriosclerosis (hardening of the arteries)

• Involved in the formation of germinal cells (reproduction).

Let's go wild!

• Watercress

• Spirula

• Purslane

• Sheep sorrel

• Rose Hips

Deficiency symptoms:

• Patients with vitamin E deficiency may show signs and symptoms of hyporeflexia that progress to ataxia, including limitations in upward gaze.

• Patients may present with profound muscle weakness and visual-field constriction.

• Patients with severe, prolonged vitamin E deficiency may develop complete blindness, cardiac arrhythmia, and dementia.

When to increase it: When consuming vegetable oils rich in polyunsaturated fats.

Processing:

Refined grains lose 80%

Roasted nuts lose: 80%

Frying in oil lost 32-75%

Preserves lost 41-65%

**Fact checker: Flatfish, butter, and fresh eggs are the best source of Vitamin E for animal-based while plant-based Vitamin E can be found in wheat germ oil, sunflower oil, and all of your nuts, seeds and oils.**

## Minerals

### Calcium

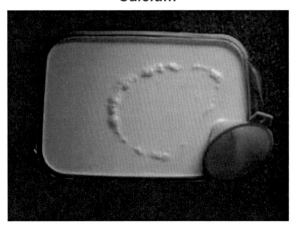

*There is nothing like fresh milk.  People think it will taste bitter or rancid, but they are delightfully surprised!*

**What is it? A mineral**

**Where is it found? Milk, dairy sesame, blackstrap molasses, beans, cabbage, and oranges.**

**What is its function?**

**Calcium is involved in bone and teeth formation, muscular contraction, nerve impulse transmission, and blood coagulation.**

**Only 20-30% of calcium in food is absorbed by the intestines.**

**Vitamin D, dietary protein, and milk facilitate calcium absorption.**

**Phosphorous (rich in meat and fish), phytate in bran, oxalates such as rhubarb, spinach, leafy greens can inhibit calcium absorption.**

**Let's go wild:**

**• Plaintain**

- **Lambsquarters**

- **Borage**

- **Onions**

- **Gromwell**

- **Nettle**

- **Lungwort**

- **Chickweed**

- **Purslane**

- **Red Clover**

**Deficiency symptoms: Rickett's, osteoporosis**

**When to increase it: Young, pregnancy, nursing**

**Processing: Minimal loss of calcium occurs during cooking.**

**Fact checker: Dairy products, sardines and eggs are high in calcium while sesame, molasses, beans and chard are high plant-based calcium sources.**

Phosphorous

**What is it? A mineral.**

**Where is it found? Phosphorous is found in both animal and plant foods.**

**What is its function?**

- **It is involved with calcium in the formation of bones and teeth.**

- **It is involved in the chemical reactions that release energy.**

- **It forms part of nucleic acids, DNA and RNA.**

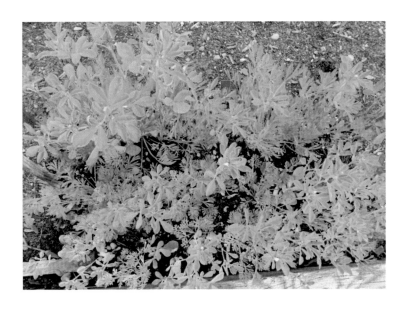

*Fenugreek is easy to grow, radio-protective and gets rid of your respiratory issues.  Bonus:  Excellent herb for cooking.*

Phosphorous is much more easily absorbed than calcium. About 70% of Phosphorous in food is consumed.

Let's go wild!

• Lambsquarters

• Fenugreek

• Oats

• Carrots

• Chestnuts

• Chickweed

• Red Clover

Deficiency symptoms: Muscle weakness, loss of appetite, bone pain

**When to increase it: Maintain a balance of 1:1 ratio with calcium**

**Processing: Very slight loss through processing.**

**Fact checker: Cheese fish, dairy are great sources of animal Phosphorous while bran, wheat germ and sunflower seeds, as well as oats and rice, are good sources of plant-based Phosphorous.**

**Cosmic ray situation: Add phosphorus to plants exposed to frequent lightning storms to offset nitrogen fixation (you need it for plants to make flowers).**

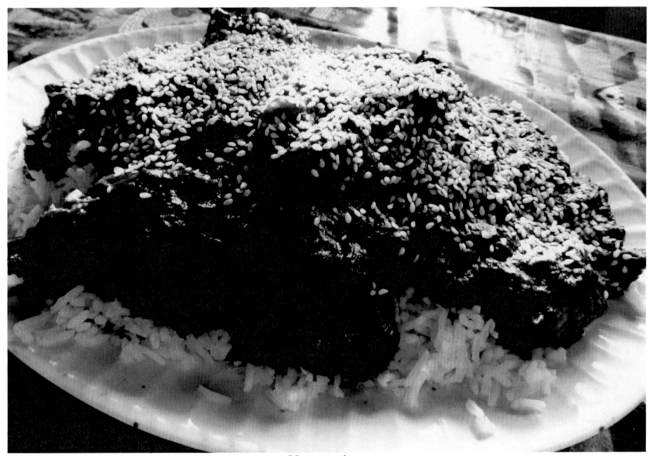
Magnesium

*Mole-Chocolate, fruit, nuts is packed with magnesium, the happy -no pain mineral!*

**What is it? A mineral.**

Where is it found? Wheat bran is the richest product in magnesium. It contains 20 times more than in milk or meat. But due to the phytates, very little is absorbed. Look to legumes, sesame, and oil-bearing nuts also.

**What is its function?**

Magnesium is involved in the formation of bones and teeth, serves as a catalyst in energy production reactions within the cells, facilitates the transmission of nerve impulses, is concerned with muscle relaxation, as opposed to calcium, which promotes muscles contractions.

• Facilitates absorption of food proteins, lactose from milk, and Vitamin D.

• Inhibits excess calcium and phosphorous.

• Excellent pain killer.

• Leg cramps, migraine headaches, muscle spasms, constipation, and especially to lower blood pressure in patients with hypertension.

30-50% is absorbed from foods.

**Let's go wild!**

• **Alsine**

• **Onion**

• **Cabbage**

• **Apple**

• **Linden**

• **Hickory Bark**

• **Purslane**

• **Milk**

• **Red Clover**

**Deficiency symptoms:** Generalized muscle spasms.

**When to increase it:** Alcoholism, diarrhea, kidney disorders

**Processing:** Very little is lost in processing.

**Fact checker:** Dairy, fish, shellfish, and beef are good sources of magnesium while bran, seeds and nuts, molasses fruit and even real chocolate syrup provides plant-based magnesium.

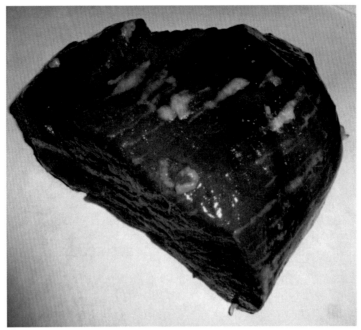

Iron

*Elk roast for corning*

**What is it? A mineral and is present in two forms in food.**

**Where is it found?**

**Non-heme iron or inorganic iron is only found in meat and fish.**

**Heme Iron is organic ad is present in meat and fish**

**What is its function?**

**Forms hemoglobin of red blood cells and cellular respiration.**

**Iron is tough to absorb through food:**

**10% from vegetables**

**15% Fish**

**20% Soybeans**

**30% meat**

**Heme iron is detrimental to the heart.**

**• Facilitates absorption of Vitamin C and calcium.**

**• Oxalates and phytates and tea tannin inhibit absorption of iron.**

**Let's go wild!**

**• Wild Strawberries**

**• Dandelion**

**• Watercress**

**• Sorrell**

**• Nettle**

**• Patience Dock**

**• Grapes**

**• Allgood**

**• Chickweed**

**• Purslane**

**Deficiency symptoms: anemia, cracked lips, brittle hair**

**When to increase it: Youth, heavy menstruation, pregnancy, hemorrhages.**

**Processing: Slight reduction in processing.**

**Fact checker: Meat, shellfish, fish are animal sources or iron, while plant-based sources include Fenugreek, spirulina, blackstrap molasses.**

Potassium

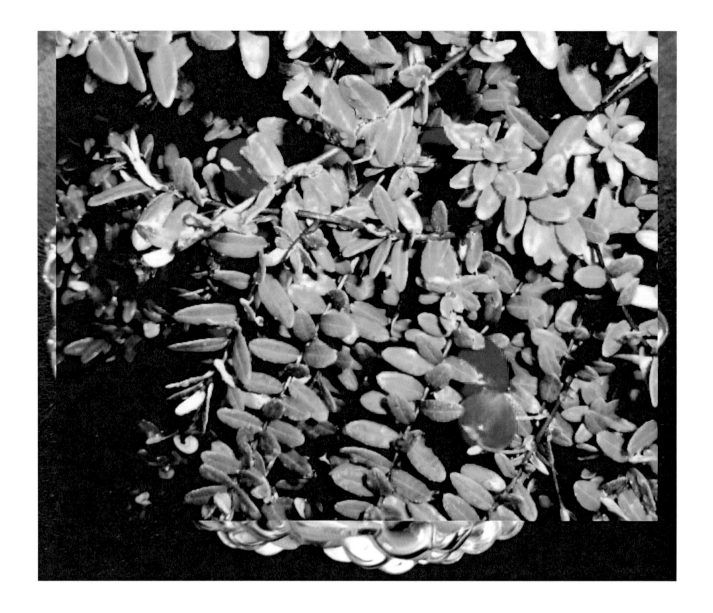

*Grow your own cranberries. There are bog cranberries and bush varieties. I love my cranberries. Their leaves turn a deep burgundy in the fall. Leave the berries on until a few frosts have passed, and they are bright red. I typically harvest the week before Thanksgiving, unless I get significant snow, then I pick right away. Cover with netting or the birds and rodents will snatch them*

**What is it?** A mineral.

**Where is it found?** It is located in both plant and animal-based foods. Bananas and all dried fruit like raisins, dates, cranberries, and prunes are high in potassium.

**What is its function?**

Potassium is the third most abundant mineral in the body after calcium and Phosphorous. The ion is the most concentrated in our cell walls. It is involved in these processes:

• **Acid-base balance**

• **Muscular relaxation**

• **Secretion of insulin to the pancreas**

• **The mineral potassium is one of the most important electrolytes in the human body. It can be used to lower blood pressure, along with magnesium and calcium.**

• **It helps muscle cramps, Charlie horses, and helps sleep if given at bedtime. It also helps with restless leg syndrome (that feeling as if your legs cannot relax and you are moving them under your covers at night).**

**Let's go wild!**

• **Asparagus**

• **Wild Strawberries**

• **Lambsquarters**

• **Storkbill**

• **Sand Spurry**

• **Wild Teasel**

• **Onion**

• **Horsetail**

• **Chickweed**

• **Dandelion**

• **Purslane**

• **Red Clover**

• **Nettles**

• **Wild Amaranth**

**Deficiency symptoms: Muscle weakness, cardiac rhythm disorders. When there is a sodium-potassium imbalance with predominant arterial hypertension is the result.**

**CAUTION: It should be given with care in patients with renal disease.**

**When to increase it: If excess salt is consumed and loss of bodily fluids**

**Processing: Slight**

**Fact checker: Salmon, cod, beef, turkey, milk, and eggs are good animal sources, while blackstrap molasses, wheat germ, nuts, dates, potatoes, grapes and melons are rich plant bases sources.**

Zinc

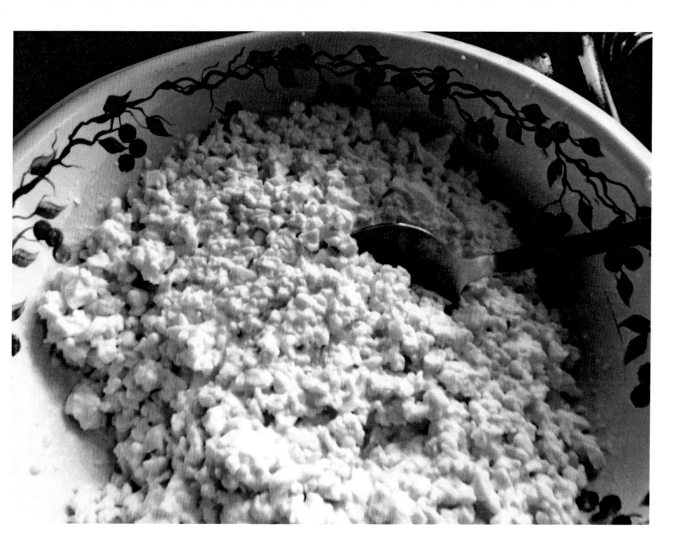

*Fresh cottage cheese takes less than an hour to make. For high yield, you need high butter-fat.*

**What is it? Trace element**

**Where is it found? Meat, oysters, cured cheese, wheat germ, sesame, maple sugar, and oil-bearing nuts and legumes.**

**What is its function?**

**Most of the zinc in the body is found in the skin, nails, hair, and prostrate. It is involved in many chemical reactions within the body since it forms various enzymes.**

**• Its primary functions include keeping the skin, hair, and nails in good condition and development and functioning of the reproductive organs.**

• Raise testosterone levels and is necessary for the production of insulin.

• There are several hundred enzyme systems in the body dependent upon zinc for their actions.

• Zinc also boosts the immune system, thus its beneficial effect upon infections.

**Let's go wild!**

• Chickweed

• Curley Dock

• Dandelions

**Deficiency symptoms:** Growth retardation and poor wound healing

**When to increase it:** Excess fiber consumption, pregnancy, nursing

**Processing:** Slight.

**Fact checker:** Oysters, meat, cheese eggs, dairy are the animal sources while plant sources are concentrated in wheat germ, sesame, maple sugar, nuts, and oats.

**Note:** Remember, if you give zinc for any length of time, you will also need to supplement with 3 mg of copper daily, since zinc will lower copper levels.

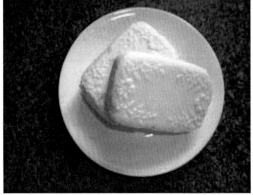

Fat

*Sweet creamery butter from your animals is the only way to get butter without flame retardants. Yes, you can make butter from goat milk. I do!*

**What is it?** Mostly triglycerides, which are glycerine and fatty acids.

**Where is it found?** Plant and animal-based food although animal-based foods, may increase your saturated fats and cholesterol.

**What is its function?** Fats act as a reserve energy source. They transport and facilitate absorption of liposoluble vitamins such as A, D, and K in the intestine.

**Deficiency symptoms:** The body can generate all fats except linoleic, and arachidonic acids found in nuts.

**When to decrease fat: Obesity, high cholesterol**

**Processing: Degraded during frying**

**Fact checker: Butter, cheeses, eggs, fish for animal-based and olive oil, walnuts, coconut, fried potatoes, avocado and oatmeal for plant-based.**

Cholesterol

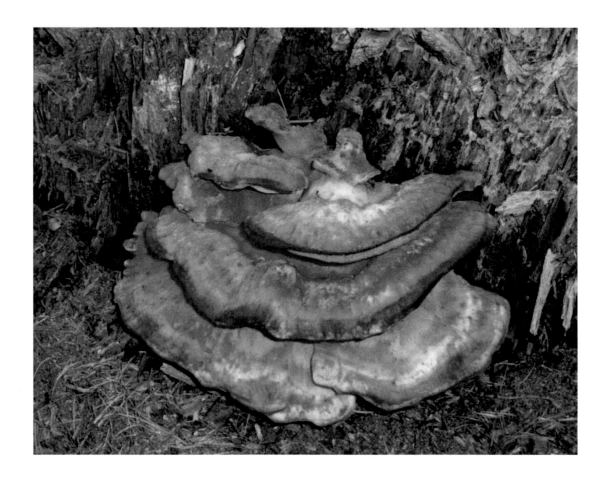

*It is such so much fun to go out into the forest to harvest Chicken in the Woods. The truth about mushrooming-know your mushrooms!*

**What is it? A lipoid (substance like fat)**

**Where is it found? Found in meats, and mushrooms. Plant-based may or may not be considered.**

**What is its function? Cholesterol forms part of the membranes that protect the cells of animals and humans. It is raw material for production of sex and corticoid hormones as well as bile, which is necessary for digestion of fats.**

**Over consumptions symptoms: Arteriosclerosis, stroke, heart attack**

**Fact checker: Animal sources include fresh egg yolks, salmon oil, whipping cream with no discernible plant sources.**

Sodium

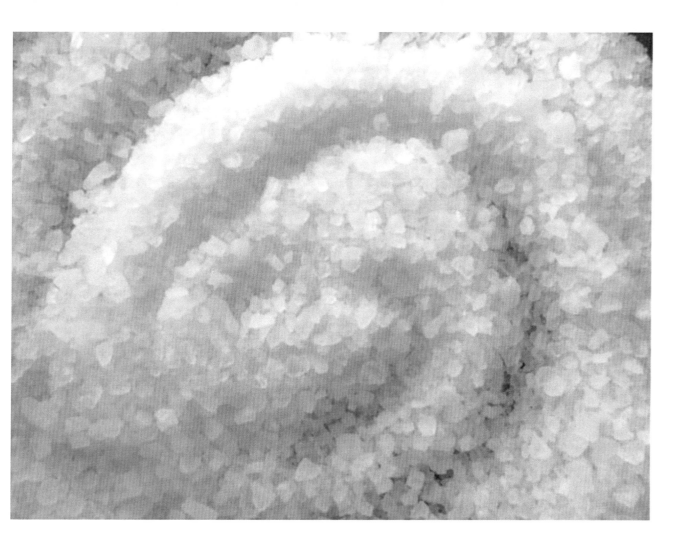

*There are different salts with different mineral contents and purposes. Gather different spices the currency of history!*

**What is it? A mineral.**

**Where is it found?**

• **It can be seen as sodium chloride, sodium iodide, or sodium nitrate.**

• **It is naturally present in plant-based foods at a low level and a higher level in animal-based foods.**

• **Hidden Salt: Can be found in processed foods, cured foods, and as an additive such as sodium alginate, sodium benzoate, and others.**

**What is its function?**

Sodium retains water and contributes to the balance of acid-base and water balance in the body. Most famous for extracellular ions.

The kidneys must eliminate the excess sodium, which tends to be 90% of the sodium consumed in food.

Excess Sodium: arterial hypertension, edema, calcium loss through urine.

When to increase it: Heavy perspiration, intense vomiting, or diarrhea.

Fact checker: Cured meats, cheeses, hamburger, eggs with plant sodium in oats, onions, potatoes, cabbage, and tomatoes.

NOTE: There must be a sodium-potassium balance.

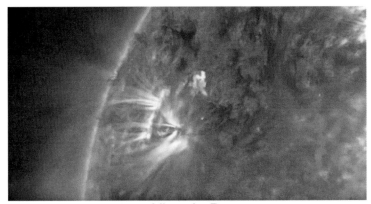
Vitamin D

*Get more Vitamin D by taking off your sunglasses for at least 30 minutes a day.* What is it? Vitamin D3 is natural, Vitamin D2 is synthetic.

Where is it found? Animal-based sources and sunlight

What is its function? Facilitates intestinal absorption of calcium and phosphorous, involved in growth and hardening or mineralization of bones and teeth.

Let's go wild!

Chickweed

**Over consumptions symptoms: Cardiac, renal, calcification**

**Fact checker: Fatty fish, liver, egg yolks, butter, whole milk.**

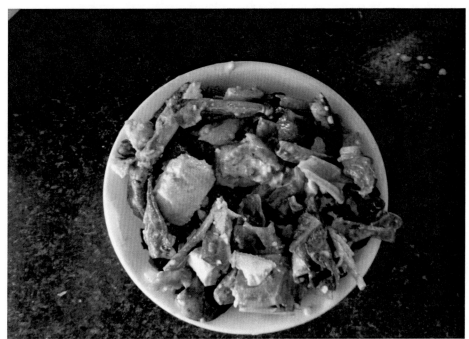
Vitamin K

*Caesar salad any way you want it!*

**What is it? A vitamin produced by intestinal bacteria.**

**Where is it found? Kale**

**What is its function?**

**Necessary for protein synthesis in the liver that facilitates blood coagulation. It is anti-hemorrhagic.**

**Let's go wild:**

**• Wild Strawberries**

**• Nettles**

**• Rose Hips**

**When to increase it: Newborns, people taking antibiotics, intestinal disorders, obstructive jaundice.**

**Fact checker: Vegetables particularly leafy greens. Animal-based food such as meat and cheese. Also, endogenous sources from within the body**

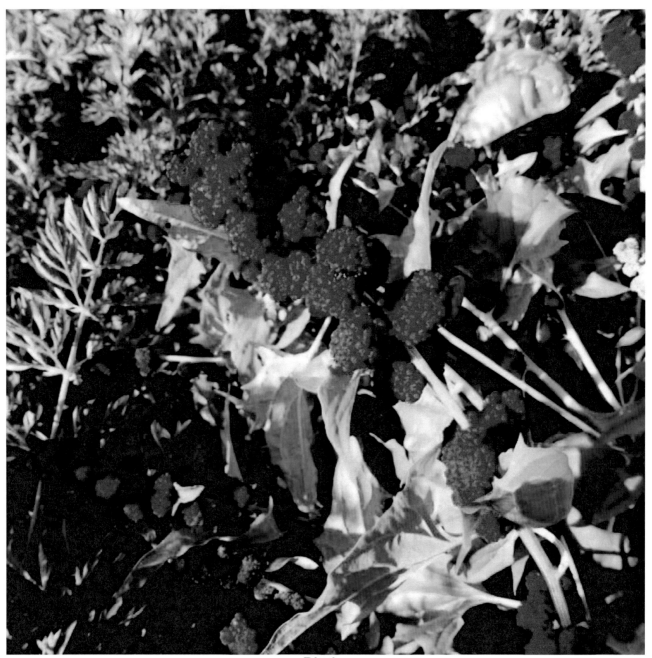

Biotin

*Are your bored with plain old spinach? Try strawberry Spinach. It is delicious and ornamental. Reseeds easily*

**What is it? Complex B vitamin**

• What is its function? Hydro soluble B complex vitamin that acts as a coenzyme in numerous metabolic reactions.

.• Deficiency symptoms:

• Rashes including red, patchy ones near the mouth (erythematous periorificial macular rash)

• Fine and brittle hair

• Hair loss or total baldness

• Anemia

• Birth Defects

• Seborrheic dermatitis

• Fungal Infections

• Psychological

• Hallucinations

• Lethargy

• Anorexia

• Mild depression, which may progress to profound fatigue and, eventually, to somnolence

• Generalized muscular pains (myalgias)

• Parasthesias

When to increase it: Certain anticonvulsants or with broad-spectrum antibiotics

**Fact checker: Found in brewer's yeast, cheese, soybean, eggs, spinach. Also endogenous sources from within the body's intestines.**

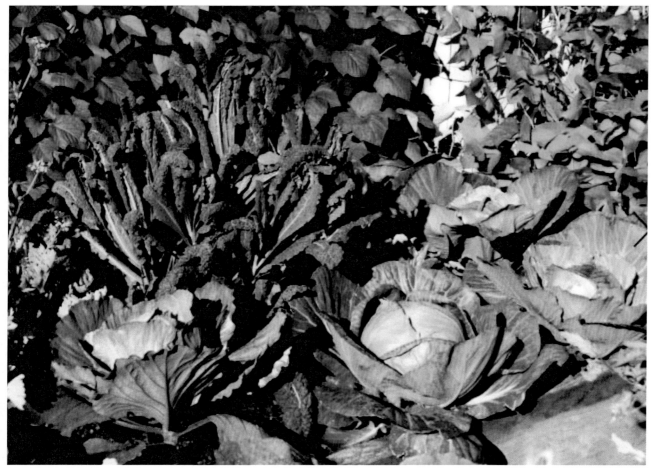
Choline

*Cabbage rules for memory preservation!  Regrow brain cels!*

**What is it? A hydrosoluble B complex vitamin**

**Where is it found? Soybeans, wheat germ, cabbage, oil-bearing nuts, eggs, livers.
The body can make some choline but not in infancy.**

**What is its function?**

**• Inhibits the accumulation of fats in the liver**

**• Involved in transmission of nerve impulses.**

**• Normal brain development,**

- Muscle movement,

- Supporting energy levels and

- Maintaining a healthy metabolism

- Detoxification

- Anti-Aging

Deficiency symptoms:

- Low energy levels of fatigue

- Memory loss

- Cognitive decline

- learning disabilities

- Muscle aches

- Nerve damage

- Mood changes or disorders

People with a condition of the liver called "fatty liver" are at a higher risk for having choline deficiency and experiencing negative symptoms. Fatty liver, also known as fatty liver disease (FLD), is a reversible condition where triglyceride fat accumulates in liver cells. It commonly develops with people who have an excessive alcohol intake, are obese, suffer with diabetes or a form of insulin resistance, and have other diseases that influence fat metabolism.

A choline deficiency may also play a part in age-related cognitive decline, including memory loss and Alzheimer's disease. This is because choline helps with neurotransmitter maintenance and, as someone ages, nerve signaling can decrease and signs of dementia can be experienced.

Fact checker: Choline can be found naturally in foods, including eggs, liver, beef, salmon, cauliflower, Brussel sprouts, and breast milk. In fact, eggs are sometimes called "brain food" because they are known for supplying high amounts of choline.

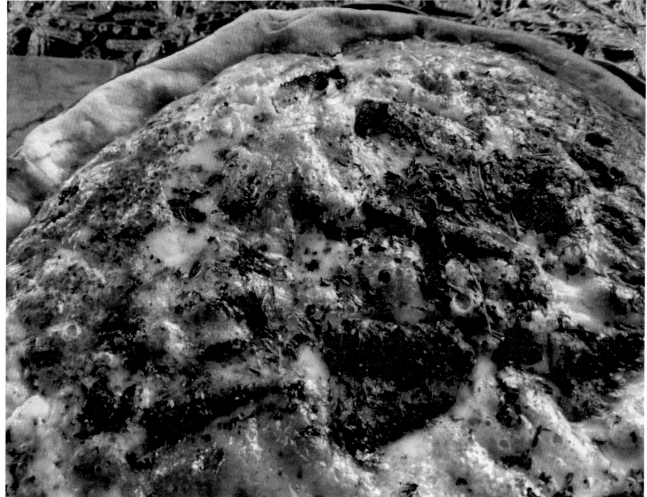

Vitamin B3

*Salmon Quiche with fresh garden herbs is a great way to get your intake!*

What is it? Pantothenic Acid or B3

Where is it found? All plant and animal foods.

What is its function?

• Synthesize fatty acids, burn them, and convert them to energy

• Produce energy in the cells through Krebs Cycle.

• **Produce antibodies**

**Deficiency symptoms:**

• **High Cholesterol**

• **Skin Lesions**

• **Diarrhea, Mental Confusion and Insomnia**

**Fact checker: Bran, whole grains, mushrooms, oil-bearing nuts, soybeans, avocado while animal-based are in salmon, fatty fish, and a variety of meats.**

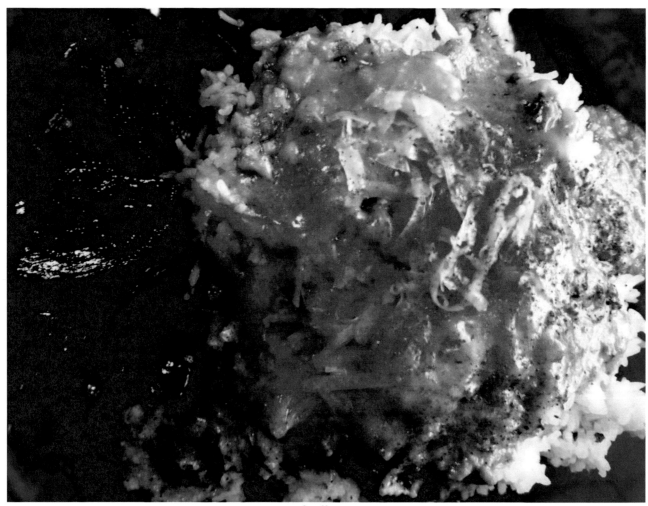
Iodine

*Salmon Au Gratin radioprotection*

**What is it?** Trace element

**Where is it found? Seaweed, vegetables grown in iodine-rich soil. Fish and shellfish**

**What is its function?**

**Trace mineral is to form part of the secretions of the thyroid gland. These regulate the rate at which energy-producing nutrients are oxidized or burned in the cells.**

**Let's go wild!**

**Nettles**

**Kelp**

**Deficiency symptoms:**

**Hypothyroidism, symptoms of which are extreme fatigue, goiter, mental slowing, depression, weight gain, and low basal body temperatures. Iodine deficiency is the leading cause of preventable mental retardation,**

Selenium

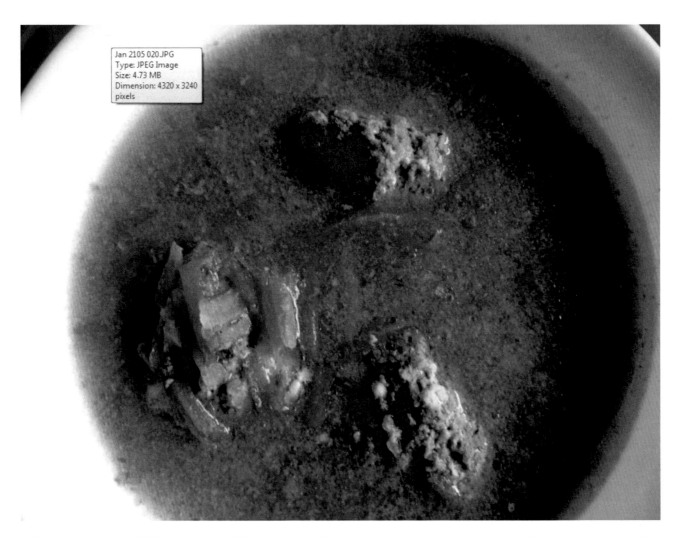

Jan 2105 020.JPG
Type: JPEG Image
Size: 4.73 MB
Dimension: 4320 x 3240
pixels

*Rosemary and Meat Dumpling soup with carrots and potatoes.  Do not overcook-30 minutes max*

**What is it? Trace element**

**Where is it found? Brazil nuts, brewer's yeast, wheat germ, molasses, or oil-bearing nuts. Present in fish, shellfish, and meat. The soil must be rich in selenium for plants and animals to have it. Most of the US is selenium deficient.**

**What is its function?**

**• Antioxidant: Acts, together with Vitamin E., Protects the cells from damage against cancer, arteriosclerosis, and degenerative diseases.**

**• Stimulates the immune system and contributes to the formation of antibodies against infectious agents.**

**• Anti-carcinogen protecting against various types of cancers such as breast and skin.**

- **Anti-asthma**

- **Fertility**

- **Longevity**

- **Thyroid Function**

- **Lowers heart disease and inflammation**

- **Boosts immunity**

- **Defends against cancer**

- **Maintains healthy eyesight**

- **Assist liver function**

- **Detoxifies**

- **Treats arthritis**

- **Treats dandruff**

**Deficiency symptoms:**

**(Selenium methionine): Essential mineral for your thyroid and your overall health. It helps reduce cancer rates when high in soil, helps boost your immune system and helps joint pain. The recommended daily dose is 200 mcg (micrograms) daily.**

Chromium

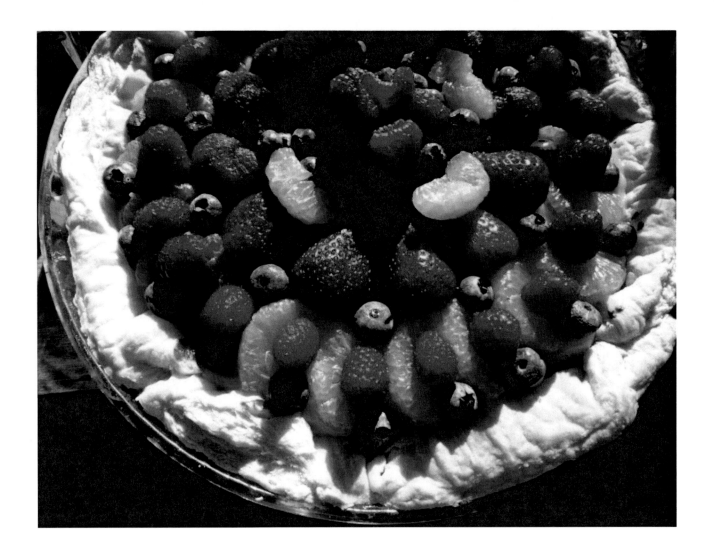

*Fresh Fruit Tarte made with puff pastry then drizzled with dark chocolate then topped with a coconut pudding. Crowned with fresh seasonal fruit and garnished with shredded coconut, if you like.*

**What is it? Trace element**

**Where is it found? Molasses, eggs, fresh fruit, wheat germ, brewer's yeast**

**What is its function?**

**Increases glucose tolerance and protects against diabetes**

**Deficiency symptoms:**

**Severely impaired glucose tolerance, weight loss, and confusion**

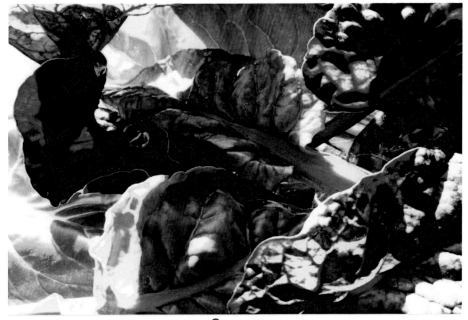

Copper

**Bright Lights Chard is sure to enlighten your day!**

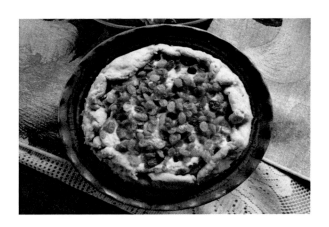

**Then try your hand at Swiss Chard and Goat Cheese or Cream Cheese Galette with an Oatmeal crust.**

**What is it? Trace element**

**Where is it found?** Molasses, oil-bearing nuts, wheat germ, brewer's yeast, oysters.

**What is its function?**

Copper is essential for the production of hemoglobin and red blood cells, as well as for the proper utilization of iron and oxygen within the blood.

Copper plays an essential role in maintaining a healthy metabolism, as well as contributing to substantial growth and repair. It is needed for the body to carry out many enzyme reactions properly and to maintain the health of connective tissue.

**Let's go wild!**

• **Wild Amaranth**

**Deficiency symptoms:**

• **Fatigue**

• **Arthritis**

• **Osteoporosis**

• **Paleness**

• **Low body temperature, or always feeling cold**

• **Anemia**

• **Brittle bones**

• **Frequently getting sick**

• **Muscle soreness**

• **Joint pain**

• **A stunt in growth**

- **Hair thinning or balding**

- **Unexplained weight loss**

- **Bruising**

- **Skin inflammation and sores**

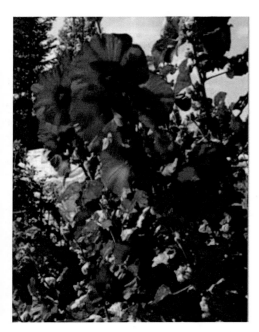
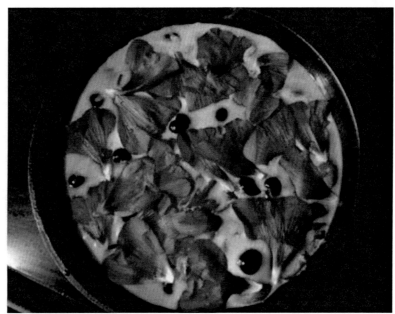

Manganese

*This is a Hollyhock and Sweet Cherry Clafoutis. Hollyhocks are hardy, eatable, and preserve well. This is a beautiful brunch idea!*

**What is it? Trace element**

**Where is it found? Whole grains, oil-bearing nuts, fresh vegetables, molasses, brewer's yeast. Present only in soils grown in alkaline or impoverished soils.**

**What is its function?**

• **Involved in formation of bone and production of insulin.**

• **Synthesis of nutrients like cholesterol, carbohydrates, and proteins. Also, importantly, manganese is included in the creation of bone mass and helps balance hormones naturally that affect nearly every aspect of health.**

Manganese is an essential trace mineral needed for many vital functions, including nutrient absorption, production of digestive enzymes, bone development, and immune-system defenses.

**Let's go wild!**

**Nettles**

**Rose Hips**

**Deficiency symptoms:**

• **Weak bones (osteoporosis)**

• **Anemia**

• **Chronic Fatigue Syndrome**

• **Low immunity and frequently getting sick**

• **Worsened symptoms of premenstrual syndrome (PMS)**

• **Hormonal imbalances**

• **impaired glucose sensitivity**

• **changes in digestion and appetite**

• **impaired reproductive abilities or infertility**

# Index

# Author Biography

**Author Information**

**For those who are actively pray for my ministry, I humbly want to thank each one of you! Last month I began weekly and special broadcasts for my Patron's in addition to my weekly articles.**

**If you consider this article informative, please consider becoming a Patron to support my work.**

**Going where angels fear to tread...**

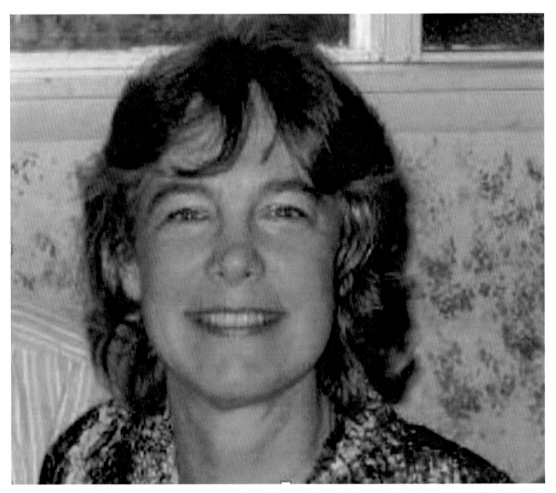

**Celeste has worked as a contractor for Homeland Security and FEMA. Her training and activation's include the infamous day of 911, flood and earthquake operations, mass casualty exercises, and numerous other operations. She also has a background in nursing-specifically pediatrics and environmental medicine.**

She has acquired an extensive skill-set in natural healing using wildcrafting, essential oils, frequency, integrated foods as medicine from her organic farm and gardens.

Celeste is FEMA certified and has completed the Professional Development Emergency Management Series.

• **Train-the-Trainer**

• **Incident Command**

• **Integrated EM: Preparedness, Response, Recovery, Mitigation**

• **Emergency Plan Design including all Emergency Support Functions**

• **Principles of Emergency Management**

• **Developing Volunteer Resources**

• **Emergency Planning and Development**

• **Leadership and Influence, Decision Making in Crisis**

• **Exercise Design and Evaluation**

• **Public Assistance Applications**

• **Emergency Operations Interface**

• **Public Information Officer**

• **Flood Fight Operations**

• **Domestic Preparedness for Weapons of Mass Destruction**

• **Incident Command (ICS-NIMS)**

• **Multi-Hazards for Schools**

• **Rapid Evaluation of Structures-Earthquakes**

• **Weather Spotter for National Weather Service**

• Logistics, Operations, Communications

• Community Emergency Response Team Leader

• Behavior Recognition

And more....

Celeste grew up in a military & governmental home with her father working for the Naval Warfare Center, and later as Assistant Director for Public Lands and Natural Resources, in both Washington State and California.

Celeste also has training and expertise in small agricultural lobbying, Integrative/Functional Medicine, asymmetrical and symmetrical warfare, and Organic Farming.

I am inviting you to become a Shepherds Heart Patron and Partner.

We live in a day and age that it is critical to be:

• Spiritually and physically prepared,

• Purity in food and water